Sexual Options for Paraplegics and Quadriplegics

Sexual Options for Paraplegics and Quadriplegics

Thomas O. Mooney
Technical Consultant,
Program in Human Sexuality,
University of Minnesota,
Minneapolis, Medical School

Theodore M. Cole, M.D.
Professor,
Department of Physical
Medicine and Rehabilitation;
Director,
Physical Disability Program
in Human Sexuality,
University of Minnesota,
Minneapolis, Medical School

Richard A. Chilgren, M.D.
Director,
Program in Human Sexuality,
University of Minnesota,
Minneapolis, Medical School

Resource Consultants
Edward Benson
LeDonna Benson
Dorothy Boen, B.Ed.
James Boen, Ph.D.
Lawrence P. Kegan, B.A.
Nancy E. Mooney
Helen Schatzlein, B.A.
John Schatzlein, B.A.

Barbara Armour
John Armour
Sandra Cole, B.A.
Jack Dahlberg, B.A.
Dan Fitzpatrick, A.A.
Bonnie Hammel, B.M.E.
William Hammel, Ph.D.
Connie Held, B.A.
Sharon Limpert

Photographers
Rohn Engh
Douglas Reynolds
Lise Reynolds
Thomas Sikes

Foreword
Alex Comfort, M.B., D.Sc., D.C.H.
Clinical Lecturer,
Department of Psychiatry,
Stanford University School
of Medicine, Stanford, Calif.;
Former Director,
Research in Gerontology,
University College,
London, England

Little, Brown and Company   Boston

Copyright © 1975 by Little, Brown and Company (Inc.)

First Edition

Twelfth Printing

All rights reserved. No part of this book may be reproduced in any form or by any electronic or mechanical means, including information storage and retrieval systems, without permission in writing from the publisher, except by a reviewer who may quote brief passages in a review.

Library of Congress catalog card No. 75-14875

ISBN 0-316-57935-1 (C)

ISBN 0-316-57937-8 (P)

Printed in the United States of America

HAL

To the illumination of dark corners

Foreword

"Hell," said a Sartre character, "is other people." Nobody knows this better than the disabled. In addition to their disability and the limits it imposes, they have the problem of getting through the heads of their able fellow-citizens that they are people with the same kinds of human desires and impulses.

The disabled *are* people, and people are sexual. Much of our sense of personhood comes from our ability to play a sexual role. The disabled share with the rest of us the misfortune of living in a society that has traditionally avoided and censured sex, but this hits the disabled harder than others. They have been subjected, like the old, to castrating black magic: "Of course they wouldn't want to talk about it; they'd be embarrassed." "It's rather unsuitable; doesn't do to raise false hopes." Generations of disabled have been hocussed out of sexual personhood by this sort of hogwash, other people's embarrassment, the pattern of institutions, and society's tendency to suppress any sex that is suppressible.

The disabled person's first hurdle in overcoming these obstacles is self-deprogramming — rejecting the idea that he or she is not a potentially sexual person and is not loveable by any person. The second is effective militancy — doing something about it. Here the most liberating strategy is open discussion. For couples with a disablement problem, the most helpful first step is discussion with other individuals or couples who share the problem and counseling of each other. In institutions, despite the embarrassment of the staff, patients should demand that the matter be talked out, that privacy be available, that sexual segregation be ended, and that disabled children be given adequate sex education and helped to realize their sexual potential. The able-bodied have projected their embarrassment on the disabled; now the disabled are learning to ignore red faces and speak out. Almost all disabled people can be made sexually functional with special counseling and a minimum of physical help. European researchers, who have seen the lives of severely disabled people transformed by the introduction of tender sexuality, are addressing most of their efforts to reprogramming people who have contact with the disabled.

Virtually nobody is too disabled to derive some satisfaction and personal reinforcement from sex — with a partner if possible, alone if necessary. When a disabled person is unable to enjoy sex, the greatest obstacle to enjoyment usually isn't the difficulty or impossibility of making particular movements, but the social convention that sex consists of putting the penis in the vagina and that all the rest of the rich range of human and mammalian sexual responses — oral, manual, and skin stimulation — are abnormal. Human sex is widely versatile and not limited to the genitalia.

A handicap more grievous and disabling than disease or injury is self-programming into invalidism, which makes a disabled person distrust his own personhood and suspect other peoples' affection as pity. Once this obstacle, as well as the others mentioned, are transcended (and this one has to do for oneself), one has opened himself or herself to an exploration of his or her sexuality. This exploration is the subject of this book. The authors suggest techniques and procedures for sexual exploration and fulfillment. In the last resort sexual expression must be tailormade for the individual, disabled or not, although the disabled have to try harder to find what works for them and how to achieve it. This is a challenge, as learning to dress oneself is a challenge for the disabled, but all Pollyannish discourse aside, the sexual challenge is probably the one best worth accepting. It has the most to do with personhood and with the full discovery that one is a loving, loveable, interacting human being — a participant rather than an onlooker.

Alex Comfort

Preface

If you are one of the 120,000 or more paraplegics and quadriplegics living in the United States today, this book can be a liberating force for you. It can help to increase your effectiveness by reducing the need to spend your energy repressing sexual urges and quelling anxieties and feelings of inadequacy. It can also be of major assistance to those in the helping professions who are committed to the rehabilitation and resocialization of adults with spinal cord injuries. In addition, this book may help able-bodied people to look again at themselves and gain a heightened awareness of their own sexuality.

In the beginning stages the purpose of this book was less encompassing. When we began to question spinal cord—injured adults about their sexuality, our objectives were to collect, organize, and disseminate the information. Material on techniques of sexual expression for paraplegic and quadriplegic men and women was either lacking or unavailable. Some could be found in brochures generated within and limited to a few rehabilitation centers. Some had been gathered by clubs organized to help disabled people. However, most of the material was available only in medical libraries, which can be used only by professionals and students in the health sciences.

This book makes information on sexual expression available to the average quadriplegic and paraplegic; here, they can find practical methods for developing sexual competence, which is an important part of human sexual expression for the able-bodied and the physically disabled alike. But more important, this book's message is its implicit sanction of the right to be sexual.

Until recently, few people have openly encouraged the physically disabled to use their bodies to satisfy themselves and please their partners. We endorse sexual expression for its ability to enhance personal pleasure, improve communication, and build self-esteem. This is especially important for those who have shunned open exchange about sexual capabilities because of self-consciousness, disability, and embarrassment. For some, endorsement may be a first step out of the isolation imposed on them by the able-bodied societal norm. For others, a major obstacle to reengaging the world in a meaningful or competitive fashion is the energy drain of feeling castrated because they are considered sexually inept. If sexual confidence can be reestablished, some will feel that they can now invest their energies in reentering the world of vocation, self-respect, and responsibility. The frank and personal language in the book also helps to desensationalize a sensitive aspect of physical disability, thus reducing the anxiety that leads the able-bodied to avoid the disabled person.

For the worker in the health professions, this book provides a source of explicit information. In the past the professional has had to rely on his own imagination or on word pictures provided by physically disabled people. Very little could be offered by colleagues. What health-care worker does not feel easier when he speaks to a client or patient from a position of information rather than ignorance?

Open consideration of the disabled individual's sexual behavior and competence does something else, too. It humanizes the disabled in the eyes of the able-bodied therapist or counselor. It helps to bridge the parent-child gap that so often characterizes the relationship between injured and able-bodied, client and professional, member of a minority and member of the majority. It is difficult for the therapist to regard as inferior a client who he knows has access to and skill with one of the most powerful of all tools of human behavior — human sexuality.

But it may be that these illustrated pages have the greatest importance for the able-bodied majority in our culture. It is they who carry the burden of societal guilt for their physically disabled brethren. They feel the uneasiness and distaste that feed on misinformation and inadequate exposure. They react in a manner that ostracizes the physically disabled from the everyday world created by and for the able-bodied.

At best, it is difficult for most of us to look at our own sexuality with an open, reassessing attitude. The task is difficult because we are uncertain about where to begin. The anxiety it evokes often serves as an excuse to avoid the task altogether. Consider those who sit conspicuously in their wheelchairs with numb and paralyzed extremities, with their urine draining into plastic bags strapped to their legs. Then consider those who have other physical problems — the fat or thin, the tall or short, the deformed or weak, the bald, those with false teeth or acne, those who are too tired, too busy, or in too much discomfort to try for sexual fulfillment. If the spinal cord—injured person can become sexually successful through a process of reassessment of goals, attitudes, and abilities, others can do the same.

We have learned that putting together a book such as this is a massive undertaking. We are grateful for the work of the many people whose efforts made it possible — for the help, ideas, and support of friends and associates who have contributed and risked so much of themselves to help others reaffirm their sexuality. Special acknowledgment and thanks are due to Nancy Mooney for her support, encouragement, and assistance with the first stages of composition and editing.

The preparation of this book was supported in part by a grant from the Paralyzed Veterans of America, Inc., Social Rehabilitation Service Grant #16-P-56810, the Commonwealth Fund, the Bush Foundation, the Playboy Foundation, the American Lutheran Church Division of Social Services, the United Methodist Church Board of Christian Social Concerns, and the University of Minnesota, Minneapolis, Medical School and Graduate School.

T. O. M.
T. M. C.
R. A. C.

Minneapolis

Contents

Foreword by Alex Comfort   vii

Preface   ix

1 Introduction   1

2 Preparing   7

3 Arousal   35

4 Intercourse   53

5 Oral-Genital and Manual Stimulation   73

Glossary   99

Index   107

Sexual Options for Paraplegics and Quadriplegics

1 Introduction

If you have a spinal cord injury, you probably have an obvious physical disability. Four out of five of you are males. You are members of the minority group of the physically disabled. You are handicapped by many things, some of which are the mistaken beliefs and myths that come from the lack of information and understanding.

Many people believe that a satisfying sex life is not possible for the person with a spinal cord injury. Fortunately, some are now finding that sexual satisfaction is possible for those who wish to seek it, whether or not they are capable of nonhandicapped methods of sexual expression. There are many ways of giving and receiving sexual pleasure.

We would like to dispel some of the myths that generally surround the sexual abilities of the disabled. In the following pages, we will share with you specific information about what some other disabled people and their partners have found satisfying, some of which you might adapt to your own method or style. We also wish to answer some of the questions that are frequently asked about the disabled person's sexual capabilities.

No one is going to think of you as a sexual being if you do not think of yourself as one. Your sexuality is your responsibility, as much as are your actions within society. What you do with your sexuality is up to you. Because of your outward appearance and your attitude toward your own sexuality, it may be all too easy for people to regard you as sexless. They often assume you do not think about, or even care about, sex. In fact, some will probably avoid talking about anything sexual for fear of hurting your feelings. Take responsibility for your own sexuality. Think of yourself as a sexual being and feel good about it. In fact, feel good about yourself. Your appearance and behavior and how you manage your personal hygiene reflect how you feel about yourself and will be communicated to those around you.

The importance of good personal hygiene for a better self-image and appealing appearance cannot be stressed enough. This is true not only for a sexual relationship but for your general health as well. Whether you can manage it yourself or your partner has to help you, it will be well worth your time to be as clean as possible.

Communication is the essence of all relationships. But for you, because of your situation, it takes on more importance. Communicating with your partner about what you can do sexually is very important. Do not assume that your partner knows what you know or that he or she will initiate discussion. Your partner might be curious about what you can do sexually or physically but might hesitate to bring up the subject.

Because of your physical problems, a clear understanding becomes a necessity for a good relationship. During a relationship, there are various stages of trust and communication. You will have to determine when is the best time to tell your partner of your problems. Do not be afraid to be honest or to talk about any problem that you may have, whether it be with an appliance, your bladder or bowels, or sexual positions that are hard to achieve. Not only will your partner appreciate your honesty, but he or she might very well think of ways to help.

You may be worried that your partner will reject you and leave if you are too honest. This is a possibility, but without a certain amount of risk, there can be no gain. Trusting and honest communication with your partner is a very good beginning. Truthfulness about yourself and your capabilities at the beginning of the relationship can prevent problems of unrealistic expectations and disillusionment later.

For the female paraplegic or quadriplegic the stereotyped role of a passive woman, combined with the sexless stereotype of a person in a wheelchair, might seem insurmountable. But if you choose to be a sexual person, it will be well worth the effort. Due partly to the women's liberation movement and partly to society's increased interest in the disabled, you, as a female paraplegic or quadriplegic, can be as active and aggressive in your sexual expression and life-style as you care to be. As men become more able and willing to rely on their female partners for strength and sharing of the complex problems of life, your strength and cleverness in solving and coping with the problems of your disability could become important assets. As a woman, it is possible for you to receive pleasure by using such methods as mentally transposing and amplifying actual sensations through fantasy, just as any male paraplegic or quadriplegic can. We will give you some ideas about what you can do sexually, whether or not you wear an appliance, and will suggest some things you must watch for to avoid medical risk. Most important, however, is learning through experimentation what pleases you most.

Whether you are a man or a woman, when you are dating and able to get out to meet people in an able-bodied society, your attitude and the image you project are very important to the beginning of a relationship, sexual or not. You can make a relationship happen, and it is your responsibility. We know as well as you do that to be a sexual person the attitudes you have to overcome present difficult obstacles. But we also know that they can be overcome. A useful way to start is by redefining your goals — where you want to go and what you want to do. This will help you to know yourself better. You will be surprised how thinking of yourself as a sexual person will affect and change how other people think of you. Do not ask yourself what anyone would see in you. Instead, let them know what kind of a person you are and what you can do and achieve. Let them see you, not the wheelchair. Take the risk of developing a relationship, a loving, caring one that grows, be it sexual or not. Life can be exciting and rewarding, as well as disappointing. Experimenting and finding your own way is as much fun as it is beneficial. So take the chance and risk something of yourself. You can gain a lot more.

If you are among those paraplegics and quadriplegics, either male or female, who cannot achieve a physical orgasm, you might ask yourself, "Why?... If I can't have an orgasm, what's the use?" It is our opinion that you do not have to have a physical orgasm to achieve sexual satisfaction. Although some disabled men and women can feel a physical orgasm or have an ejaculation, others, depending upon the extent and location of their injuries, cannot. Some may remember the physical sensation that they had before their injury and mentally recreate and intensify the feeling to enjoy a mental orgasm. Others who were injured before they were old enough to experience an orgasm, fantasize one and report that they believe it is as good as a "normal" one would be.

If you are a paraplegic or quadriplegic male, what can you expect in the way of reproductive capability? Your testicles may be chronically infected as a result of urinary infections or long-term use of a catheter. Also, your paralysis influences your body's ability to control the temperature in the scrotum, or testicular sac. These two conditions may so damage the testicles that they become scarred and can no longer produce sperm. However, the spinal cord injury does not lower your body's ability to manufacture normal sex hormones and, depending on the level of injury, does not affect your ability to achieve a reflex erection. If you are unable to come (ejaculate, or discharge sperm), you are for all practical purposes infertile. Some doctors have experimented with other methods of obtaining sperm for purposes of fertilizing a woman (see *fertility* in the Glossary). You may want to ask your doctor about the possibilities if you are interested.

If you are a woman with a spinal cord injury, it may have caused changes in your reproductive function. However, the changes are usually only temporary and do not limit your ability to become pregnant, carry the baby in your uterus, or give birth. Your body will continue to produce female sex hormones normally. However, there is about a 50 percent chance that your menstrual periods will stop for a short time after your paralysis. They may start again within six months after your injury. Cramps associated with your periods, if present before your injury, will not return if your injury has caused loss of sensation. There will be no interference with your ability to ovulate or expel the egg from your ovary into your uterus. You will be just as capable of becoming pregnant and having a normal baby as you were before your spinal cord injury. You will also be just as capable of carrying a baby in your uterus as you were before your paralysis. However, your spinal cord injury causes certain problems of which you should be aware (see *pregnancy* in the Glossary).

Today very few people would expect conception to be the sole purpose of adult human sexual activity. Still, the ability to impregnate or to conceive is extremely important to some people. Whether or not the man can fertilize the woman or the woman can bear children remains a measure of personhood and is an important dimension of human sexuality to some.

There are some paraplegics and quadriplegics who believe that, because of their disability, they cannot expect to receive much enjoyment from sex and that the only satisfaction they can hope for is the pleasure they receive from satisfying their partners. While this may be a noble attitude, you cannot maintain it for very long before you begin to feel left out. Your sex life may slow down until finally you and your partner stop having sex altogether. It is important to give pleasure and satisfy your partner, but it is also essential that you too receive pleasure. In fact, for good sexual expression, there should be a balance of sexual give-and-take between the two people involved. If either you or your partner thinks that the sexual relationship is one-sided, the guilt and animosity that result can affect your relationship and make you both disappointed or even miserable.

Sensory amplification, the method used by some disabled men and women to achieve the most pleasure and satisfaction from a sensory input, is the act of thinking about a physical stimulus, concentrating on it, and amplifying the sensation in your mind to an intense degree. Thus, it is possible to achieve a higher level of satisfaction and possibly a mental orgasm. Some who have lost physical sensation in the genital area substitute or transfer a sensation from an area of the body that has retained some feeling, such as the inside of an arm, the neck, breasts, buttocks, or around the anal area. By transposing these sensations mentally or by using your imagination to create a fantasy, you may find intense satisfaction.

Many paraplegics and quadriplegics feel it is necessary to be able to see their partner's reactions. Feeling or watching your partner's reactions to what you are doing lets you know that you are pleasing him or her. That knowledge may heighten your own satisfaction and pleasure. There are some who have such a great ability to fantasize and such good empathy with their partners that they can "feel" what their partners are feeling.

There is something you should watch out for if you have an injury above the fourth thoracic vertebra. During intercourse, or when nearing a climax or orgasm, you could experience a very painful headache. *Autonomic hyperreflexia* is the medical term for this reaction. What is happening is that your blood pressure rises very high — high enough to cause the headache. There are other causes for this type of headache, but if it happens during intercourse or masturbation, stop and rest before continuing. This will allow your blood pressure to fall and your headache to disappear.

In succeeding chapters, we hope to offer you, as a handicapped person, a better idea of the possibilities and the sexual options that are available for a more satisfying sex life. We will present several aspects of sexual activity such as preparation, turn-ons, foreplay, pleasuring, how to achieve and maintain a reflex erection of the penis, positions for intercourse, oral-genital sex, and manual stimulation. We will also discuss which options can be used without creating new problems or aggravating existing medical conditions of your particular disability. The ideas we will suggest are some that other paraplegics and quadriplegics have used very successfully for sexual expression. In presenting these suggestions, however, we make the following assumptions:

1. Whatever seems satisfying and pleasurable to a couple is acceptable as long as they mutually agree.
2. It is important for people to experiment and discover what is satisfying.
3. It is important for couples to communicate to each other what they have found pleasing and satisfying.

When couples follow these precepts, we believe they find that sexuality can be a healthy and important part of their lives, whether or not a physical disability exists.

2 Preparing

It is unfortunate that there are no magic words that will get you ready, undressed, and into position in the blink of an eye (1). However, some forethought and discussion with your partner about the necessary mechanics can make getting ready and into bed a turn-on for both of you. As we have said, cleanliness is important to anyone's sexuality, but especially to people who have to wear catheters or devices to collect urine (2). Often, just before sexual activity, it is helpful to go into the bathroom and prepare by cleaning up (3, 4, 5).

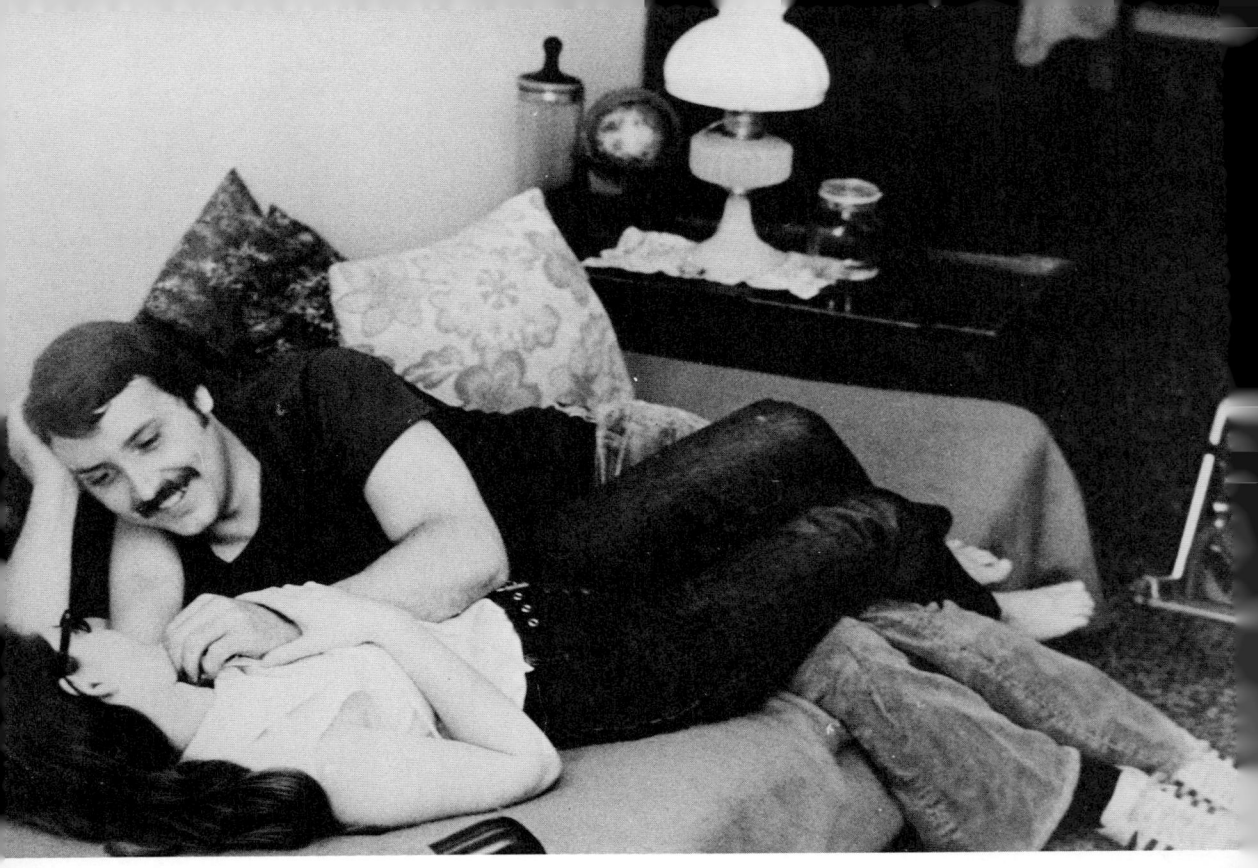

1

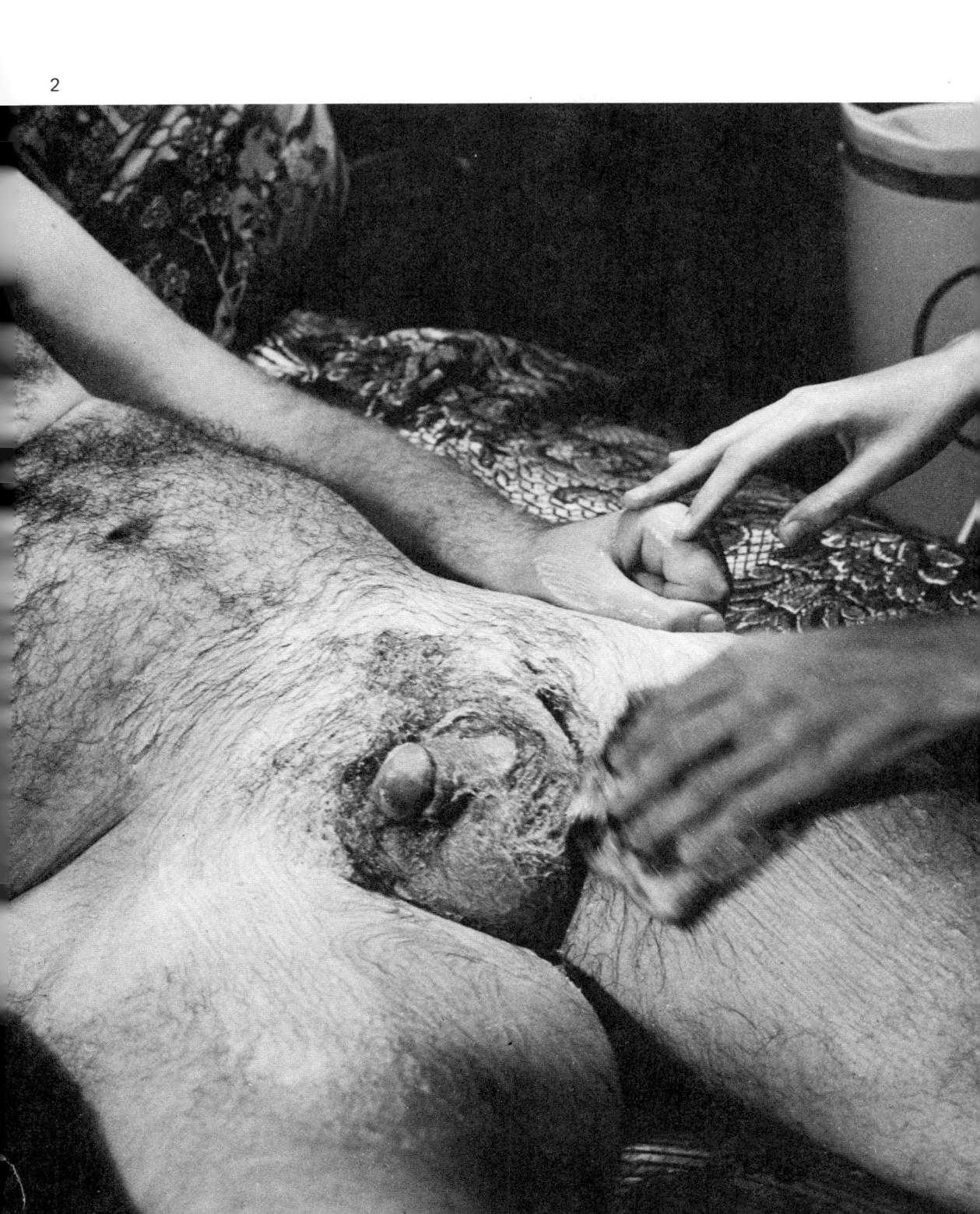

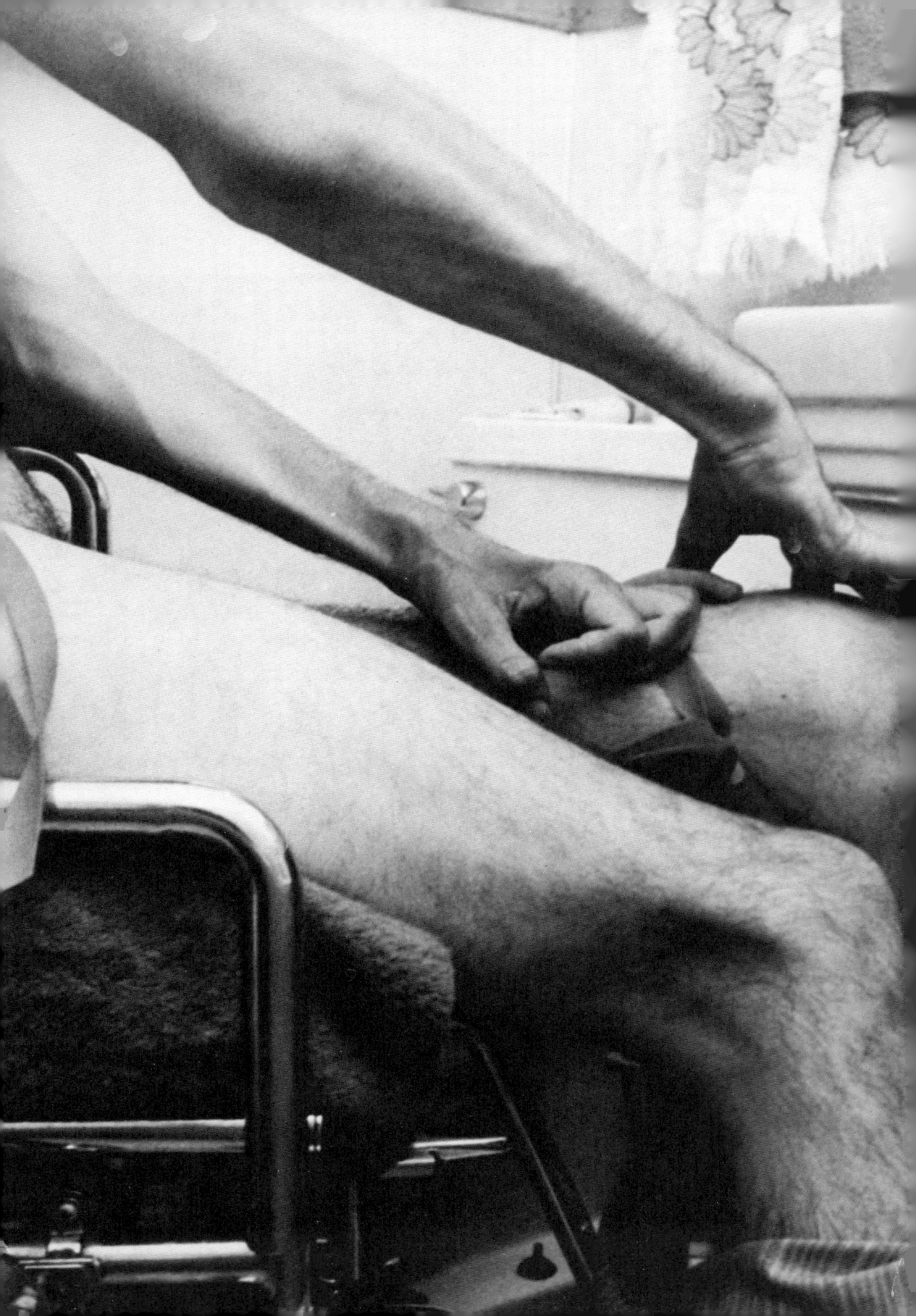

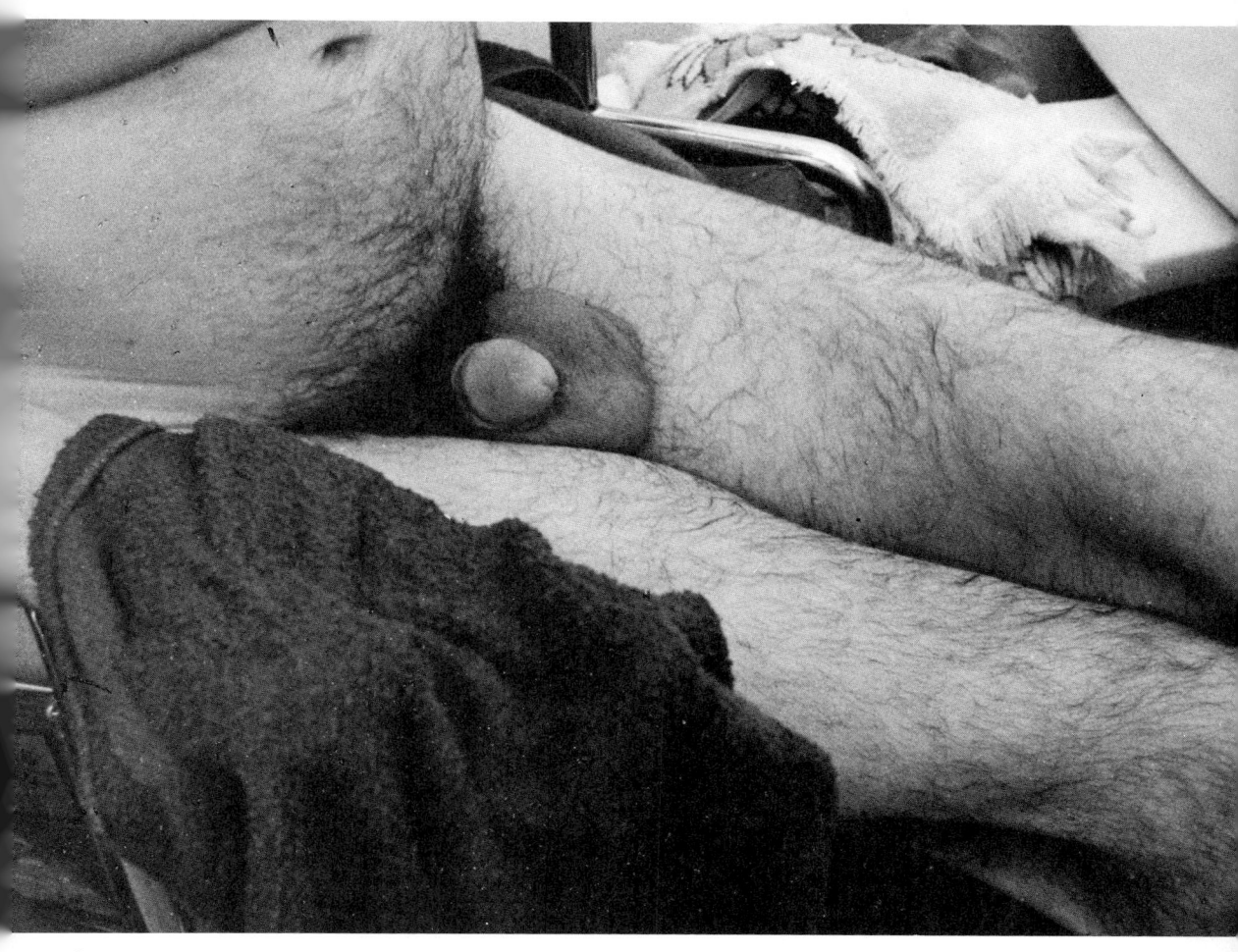

4

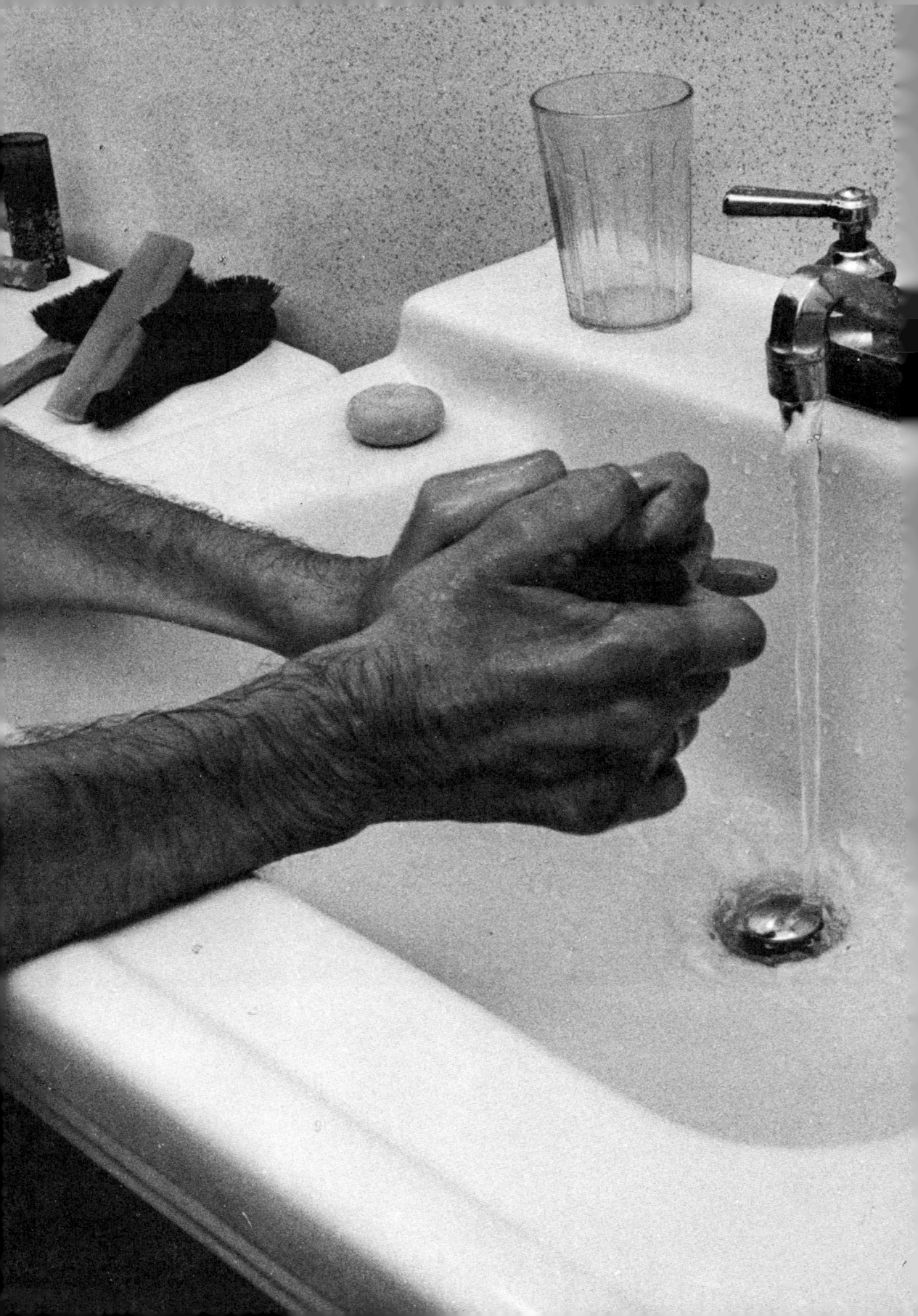

5

It is not always necessary to remove the catheter from the penis before attempting intercourse. The catheter may be bent and folded over along the shaft of the penis where it will be out of the way (6). However, take care not to anchor it down while the penis is still soft. It should be allowed to slide in the penis as erection is taking place. The reason for this is that many catheters have balloons at the end which is inside the bladder. An erection could pull the balloon out of the bladder and into the outflow tube (urethra) producing stretching and bleeding. The penis and the catheter are easily accommodated by the woman's vagina in this position and should cause no irritation to her.

6

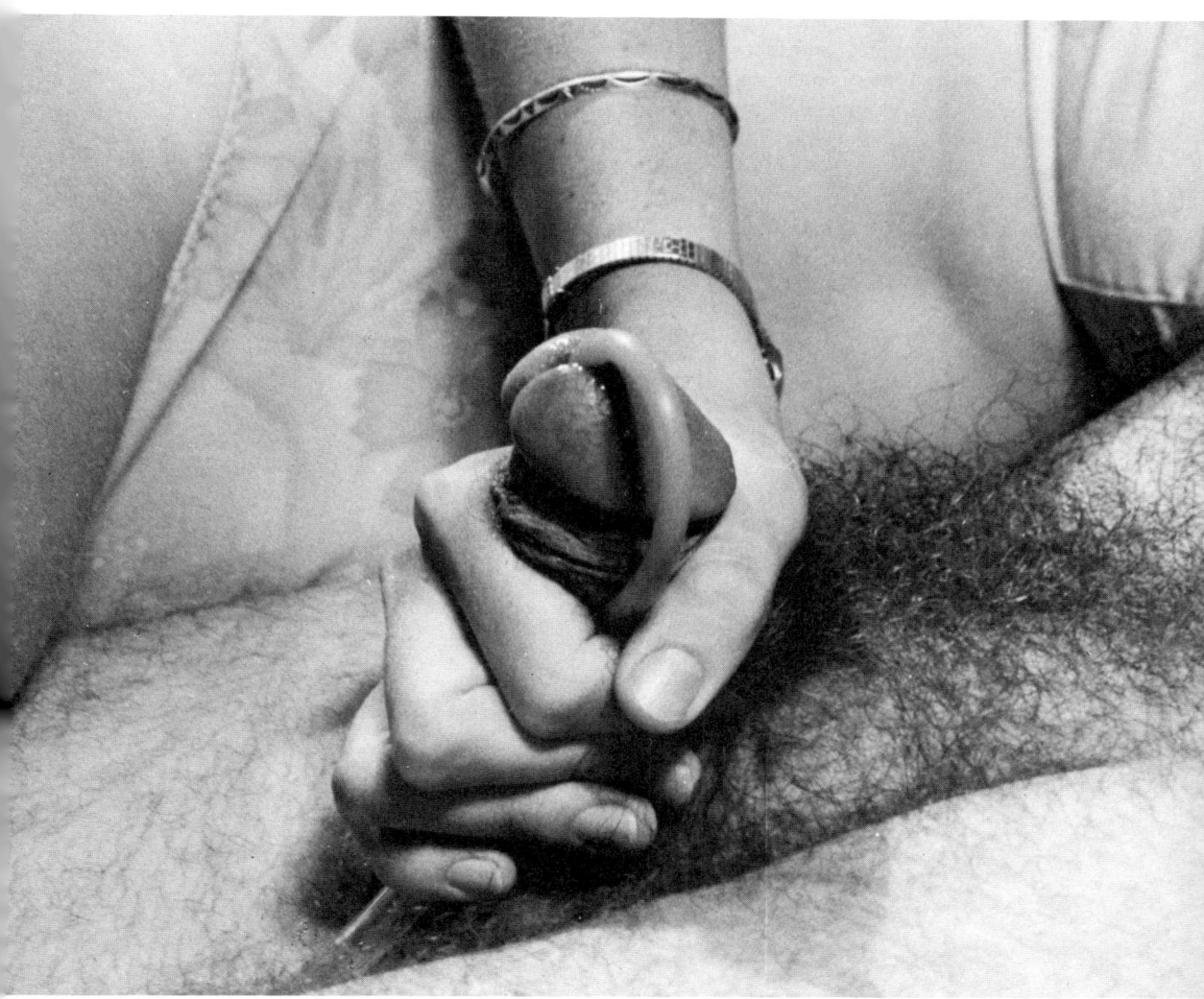

In the case of a female paraplegic or quadriplegic, the catheter can also be pushed aside and positioned out of the way. Both the male and female should use enough caution so that the action of intercourse does not pull the catheter out of the bladder. Almost any lubricant (except petroleum jelly, which gets sticky) can and should be used when the catheter is in place. This method works well unless rubbing against the catheter causes some discomfort for your partner.

For those who have had an ileostomy, the urine-collection bag may produce some positioning problems. These can be solved by emptying the bag and leaving it on or by attaching a drainage tube from the bag to a drainage bottle.

Once the tube or bag is positioned out of the way, your partner may find that he or she will want to modify some positions in order to avoid sitting or lying on the bag or tubing and cutting off the flow of urine (7). Urine-collection bags and tubes need not stand in the way of physical intimacy if reasonable care is taken to position them (8, 9). Adhesive tape around the seal of the diversion bag will help if you are afraid of breaking the seal when your activity becomes strenuous. Your partner can help to avoid leakage of your urine-collection device by being careful to avoid chafing, rubbing, or pressing against it (10). During nighttime use, a longer tube connecting the urine-drainage bag to a larger bottle at the bedside precludes having to awake at night to empty the smaller leg bag (11).

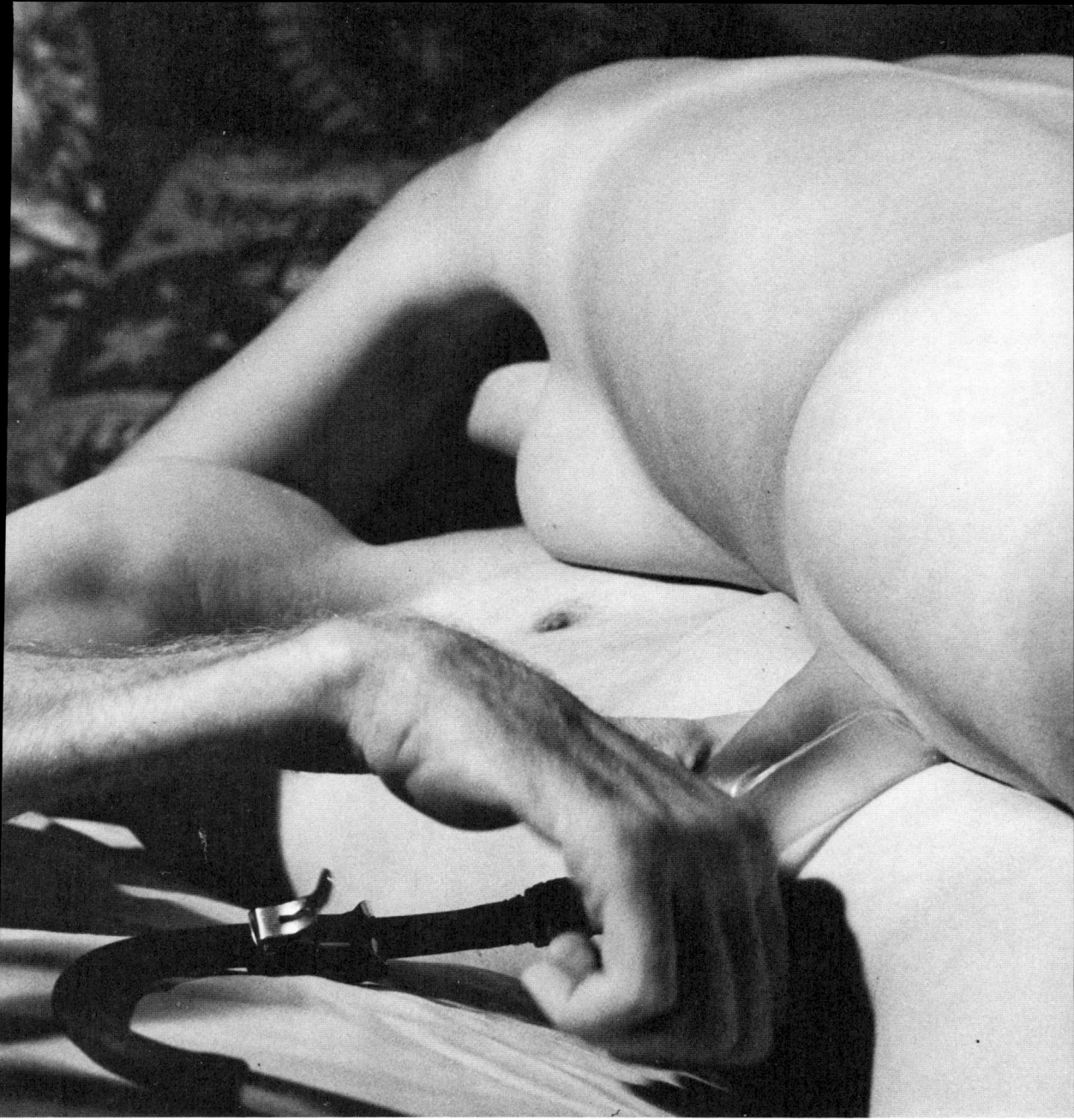

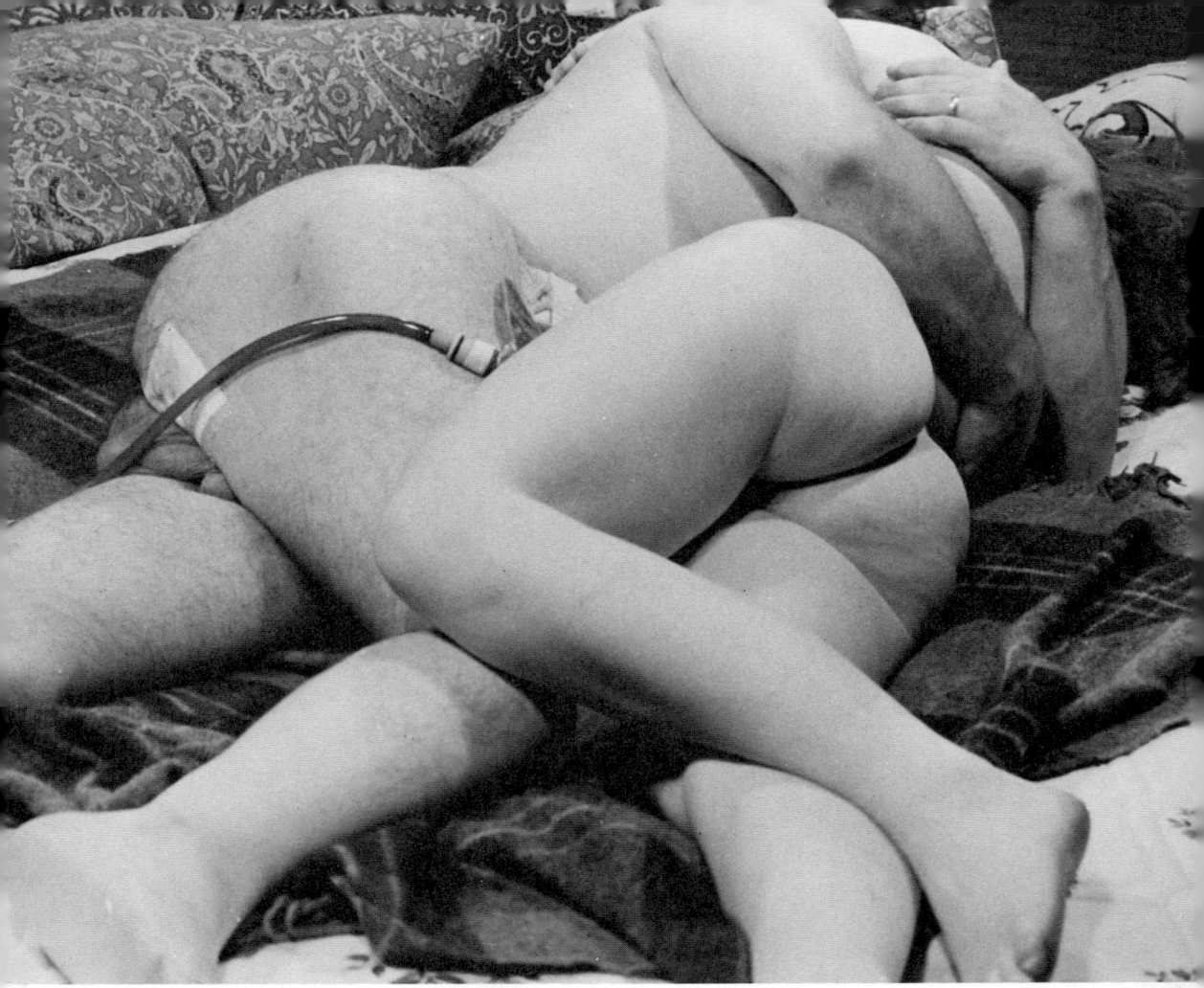
8

9

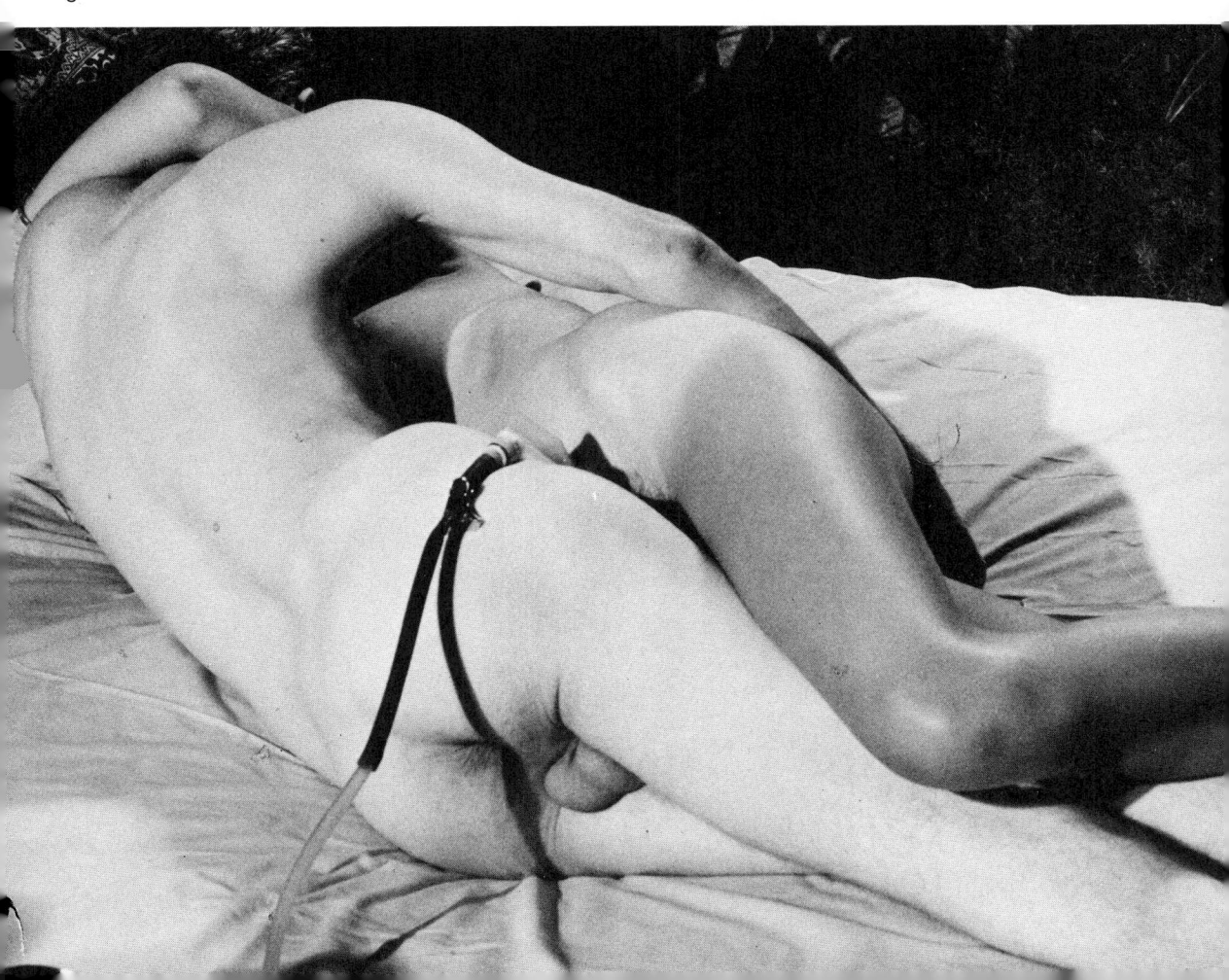

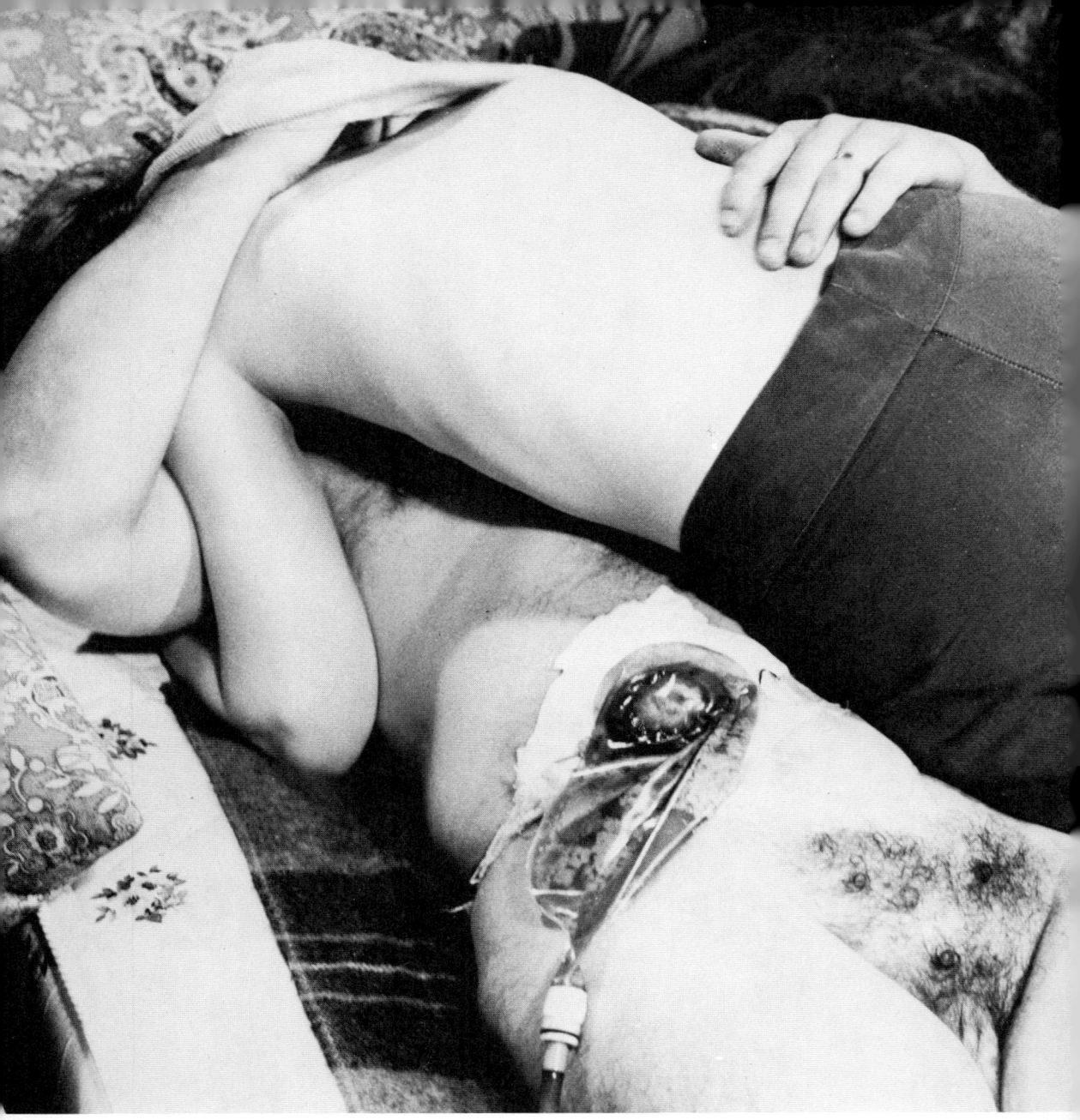
10

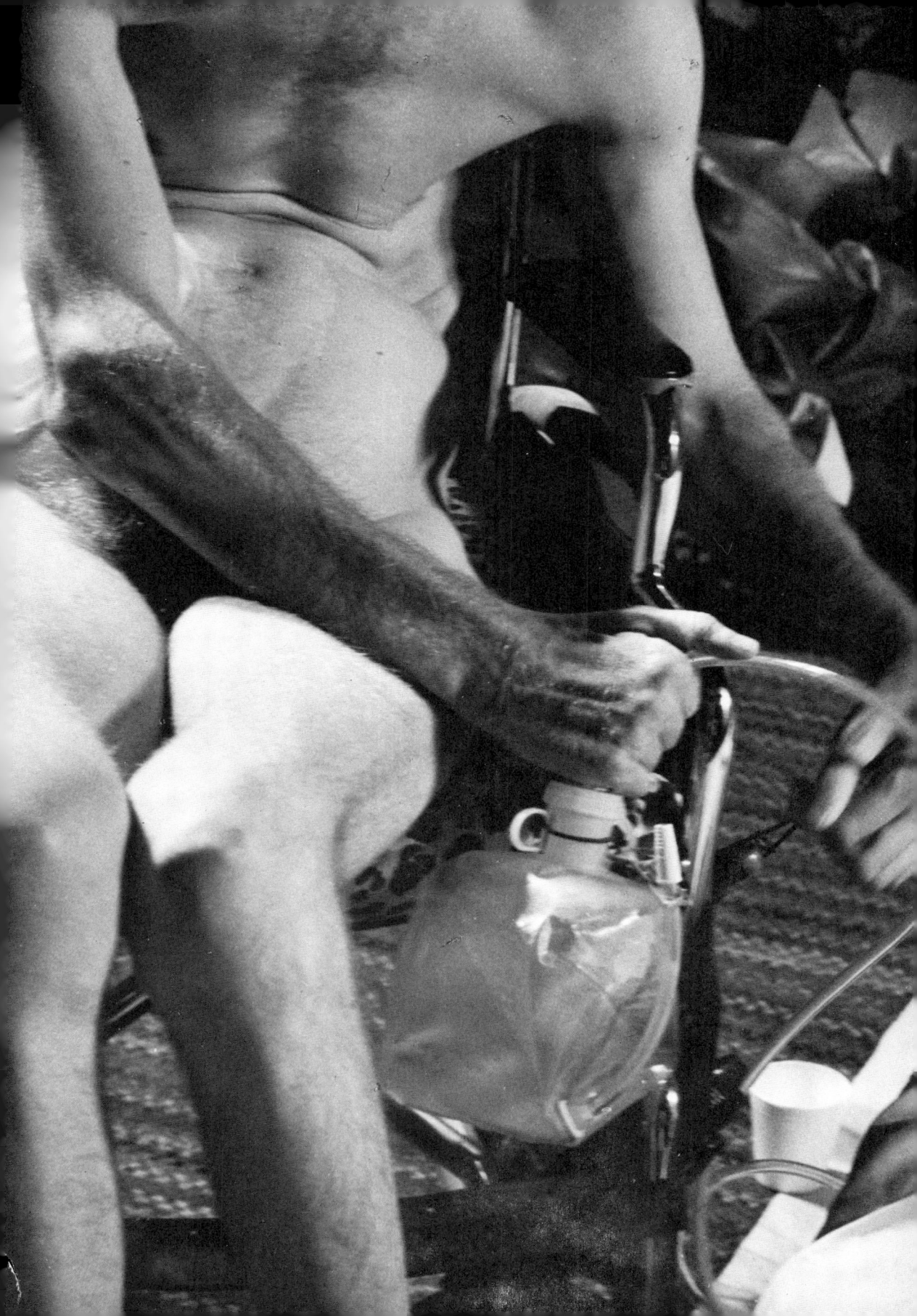

The external or condom type of urinary drainage appliance, sometimes called the *Texas catheter* (or gizmo, rig, and so on), can be removed. It is really no more difficult to remove before sex than it is to remove underwear (12).

12

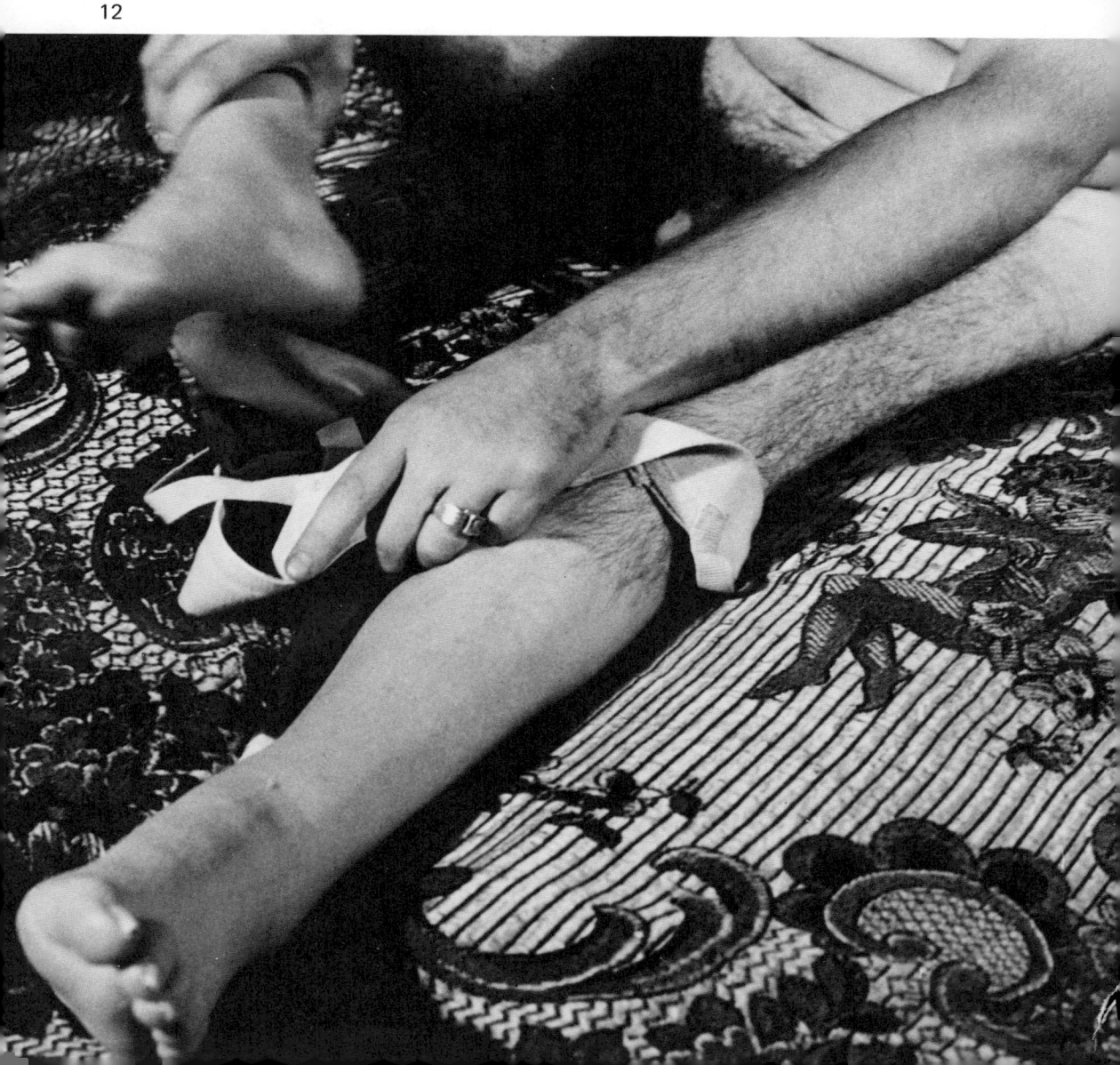

If your bladder is likely to leak or empty itself during sexual activity, it is often wise to apply Credé's method, or hand pressure over the bladder, to empty it before beginning your sexual activity (13). After using Credé's method or another method of emptying the bladder, you are pretty much unhampered until the bladder fills again and contracts. It is a good idea to keep a urinal, bottle, or can by the bed.

13

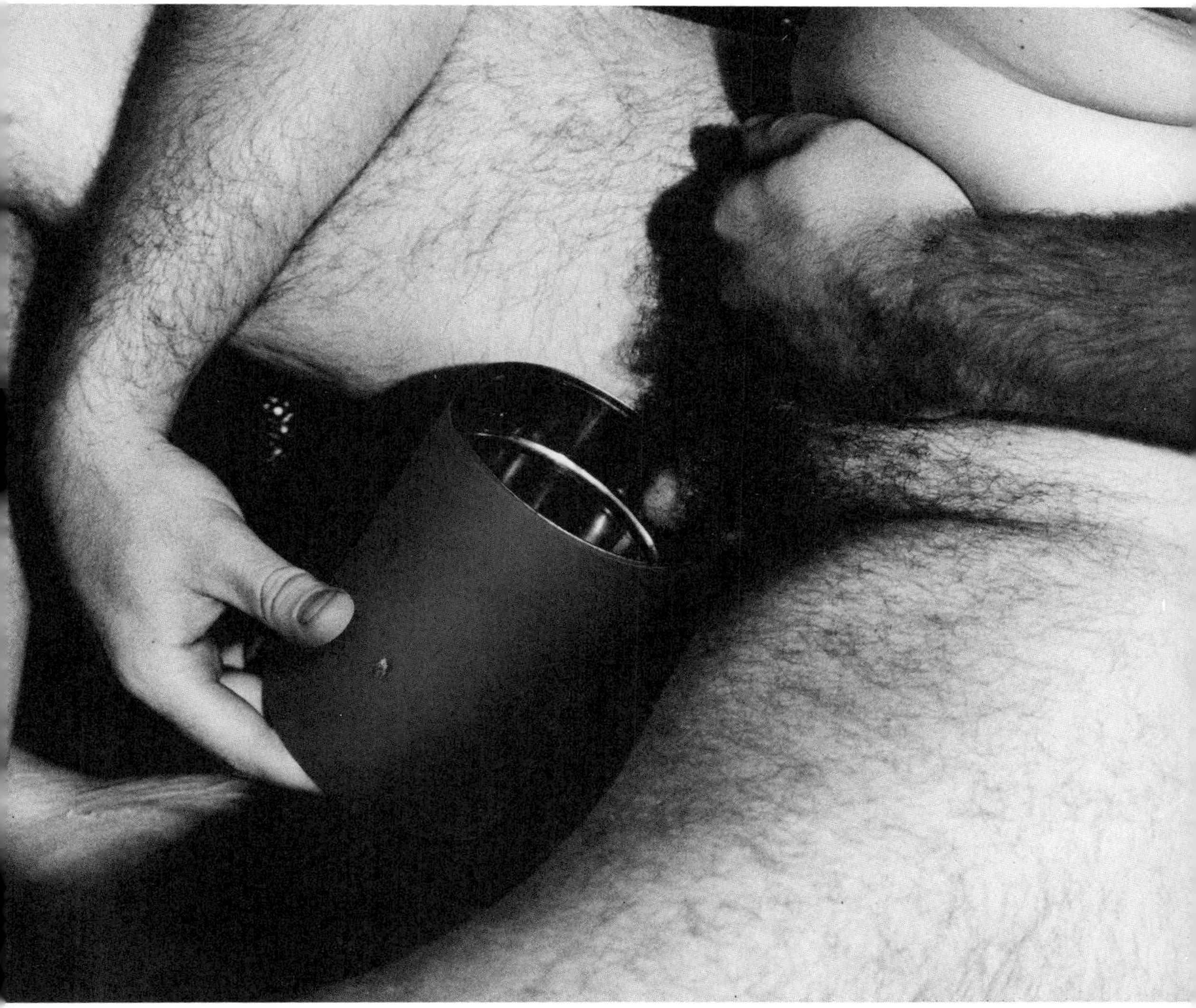

If you and your partner do not wish penile-vaginal contact, the appliances can be emptied, left on, and attached to a drainage bottle. You will then be fairly unencumbered to enjoy some of the other options of sexual expression.

A Texas catheter connected to a short tube and leg bag is shown in photograph 14, and one connected to a long tube and nighttime drainage bottle is shown in 15.

14

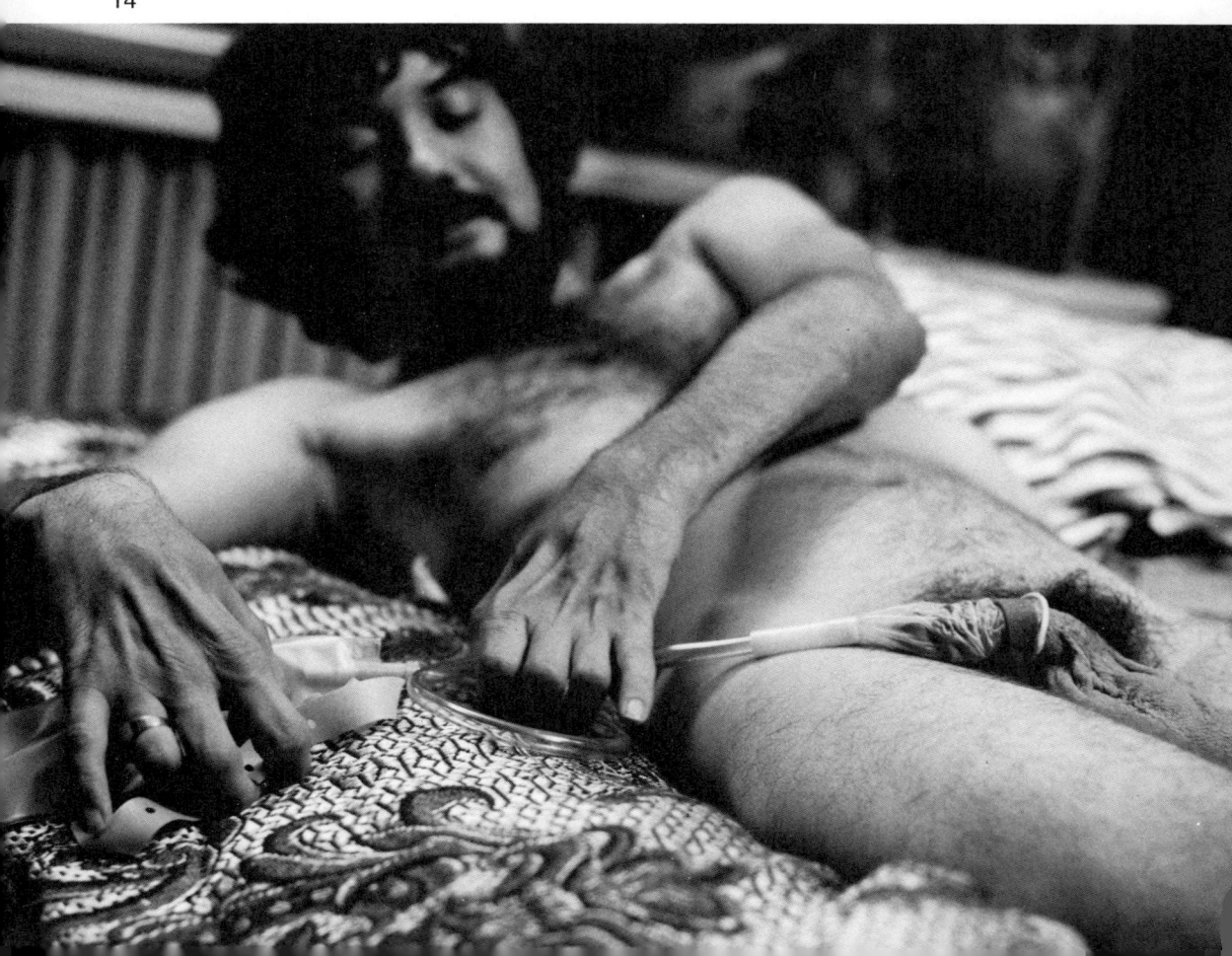

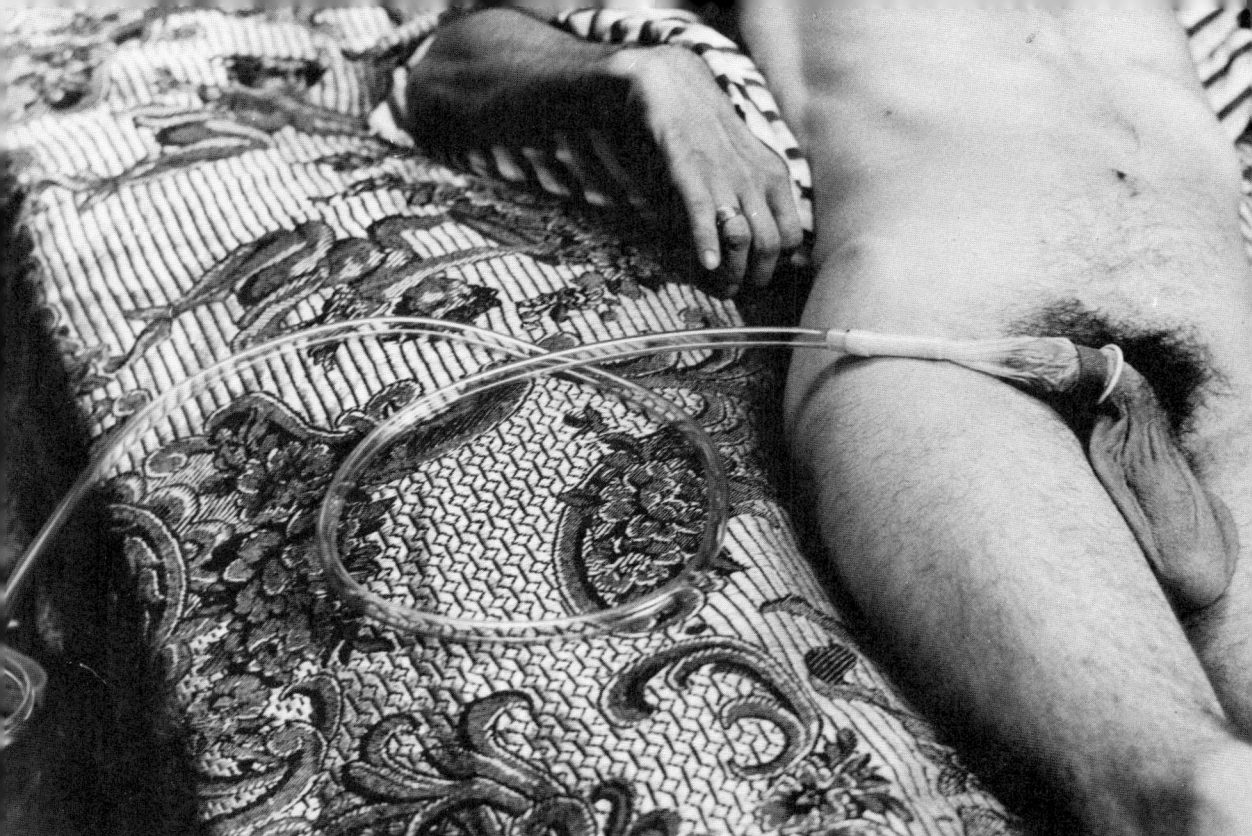

15

In any of the positions in which your catheter is attached to a drainage bottle, a little care must be taken to keep the urine flowing freely and the appliances from kinking. Otherwise, you and your partner might have to pause in your lovemaking to dry off and make repairs. If it has been your experience to have urinary leakage during sexual activity, it may be wise to bring a towel to bed with you so that leakage can be dealt with immediately and does not cause delays or embarrassment (16).

Although leakage is an inconvenience, it is not a catastrophe. Your partner should be told that leakage is possible. It is our experience that when a partner is informed about the possibility of accidents of this nature, he or she is almost always very understanding and is not over-concerned when it happens (16).

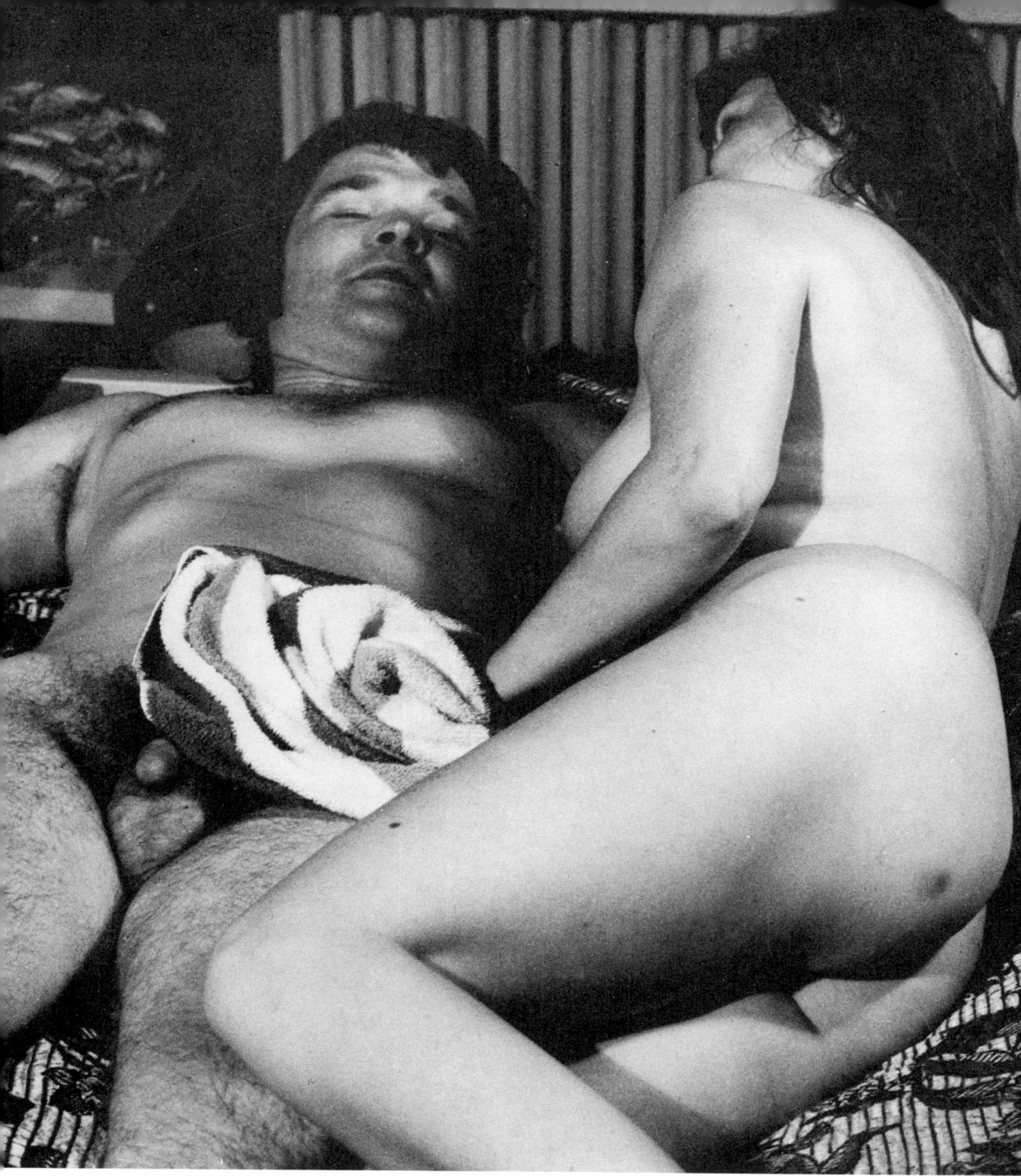

There are times when a quick check of connectors and drainage tubing is an inconvenience: for example, when the male partner checks a connector as the female partner continues to insert his penis into her vagina (17).

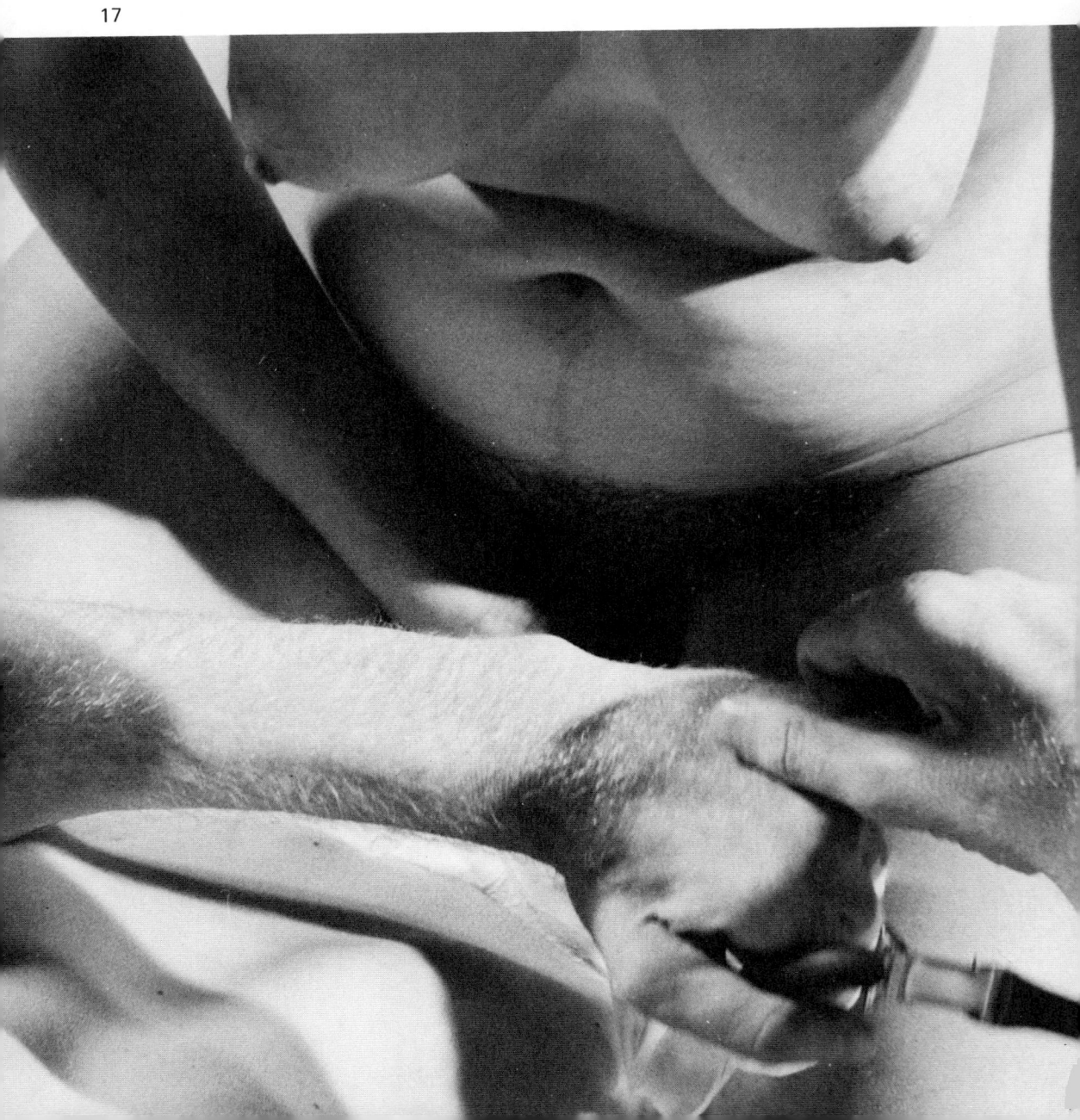

17

In some instances it may be necessary for your partner to help you in preparing. For instance, if it is difficult for you to maintain your balance while sitting on a soft bed, your partner may be able to help by providing a backrest for you while you undress or remove an appliance (18).

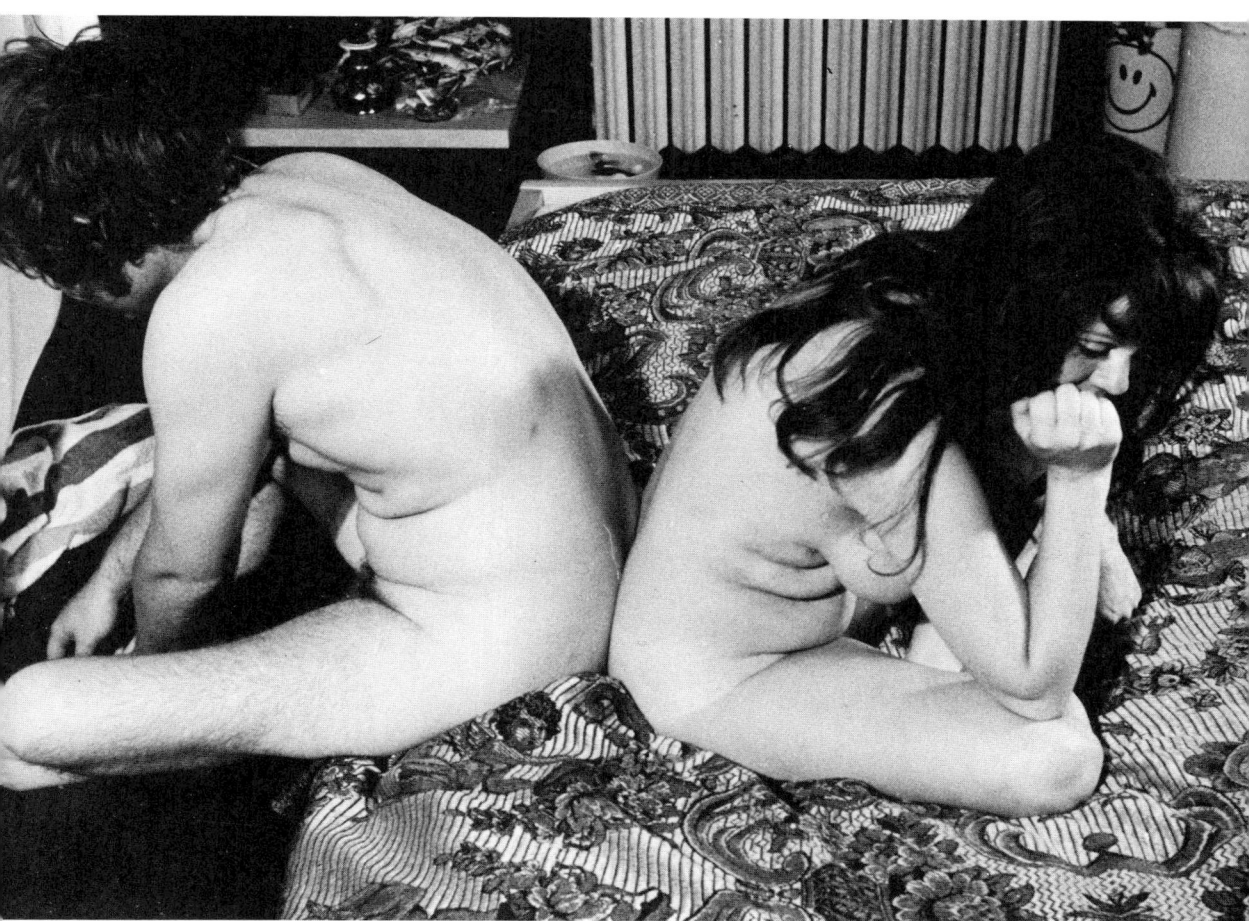

If your injury is such that you are unable to help much in getting ready, and your partner is unable to manage alone, there are still other options available. An aide or some other third person can help attach any appliances and assist in the transfer from chair to bed. Although this method may concern you and your partner because of a lack of privacy and the inconvenience of having a third person involved in your sex life, the extra efforts in talking it out will facilitate deeper understanding.

Quadriplegics with weakened hands and fingers sometimes must ask for help from their partner or an attendant. A woman can assist her partner in putting on a condom (Texas) catheter (19). In photograph 20, an able-bodied male attendant is deflating the balloon at the end of a Foley catheter that is being removed for purposes of intercourse and afterward will be reinserted in a sterile manner. Before sexual activity the catheter can be easily removed by a trained attendant. Its insertion requires strict adherence to sterile technique (21), which can be taught to you by your doctor or nurse.

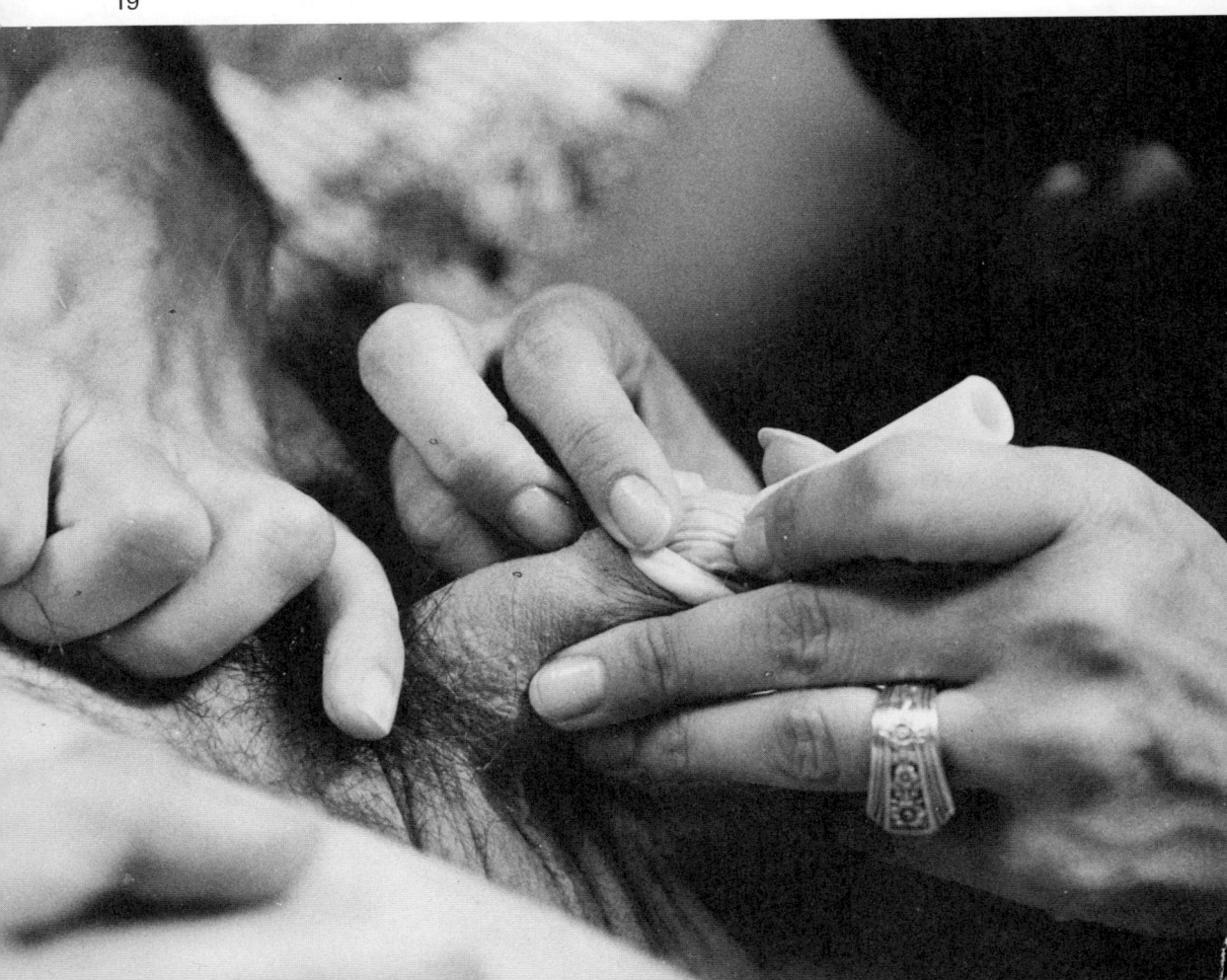

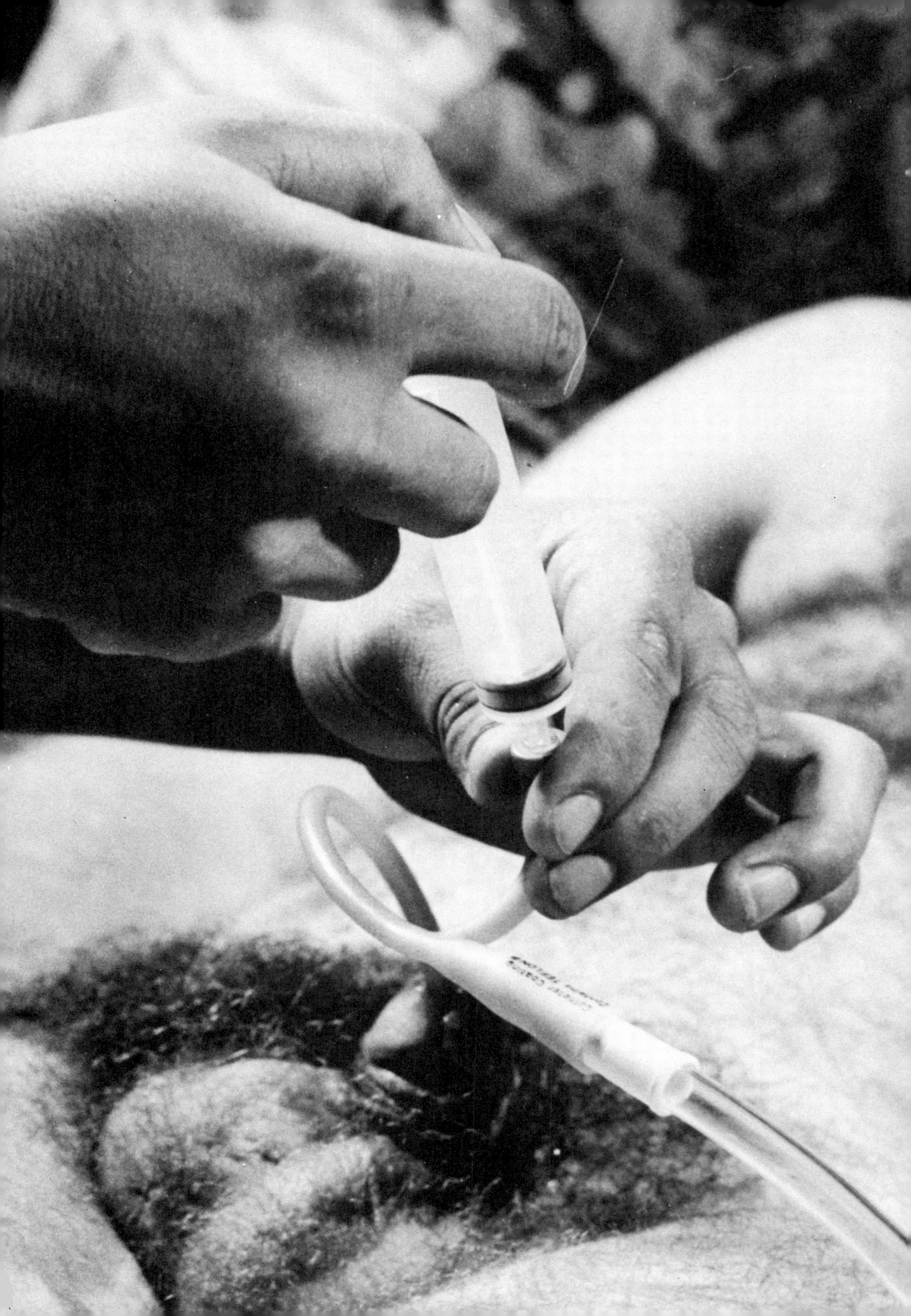

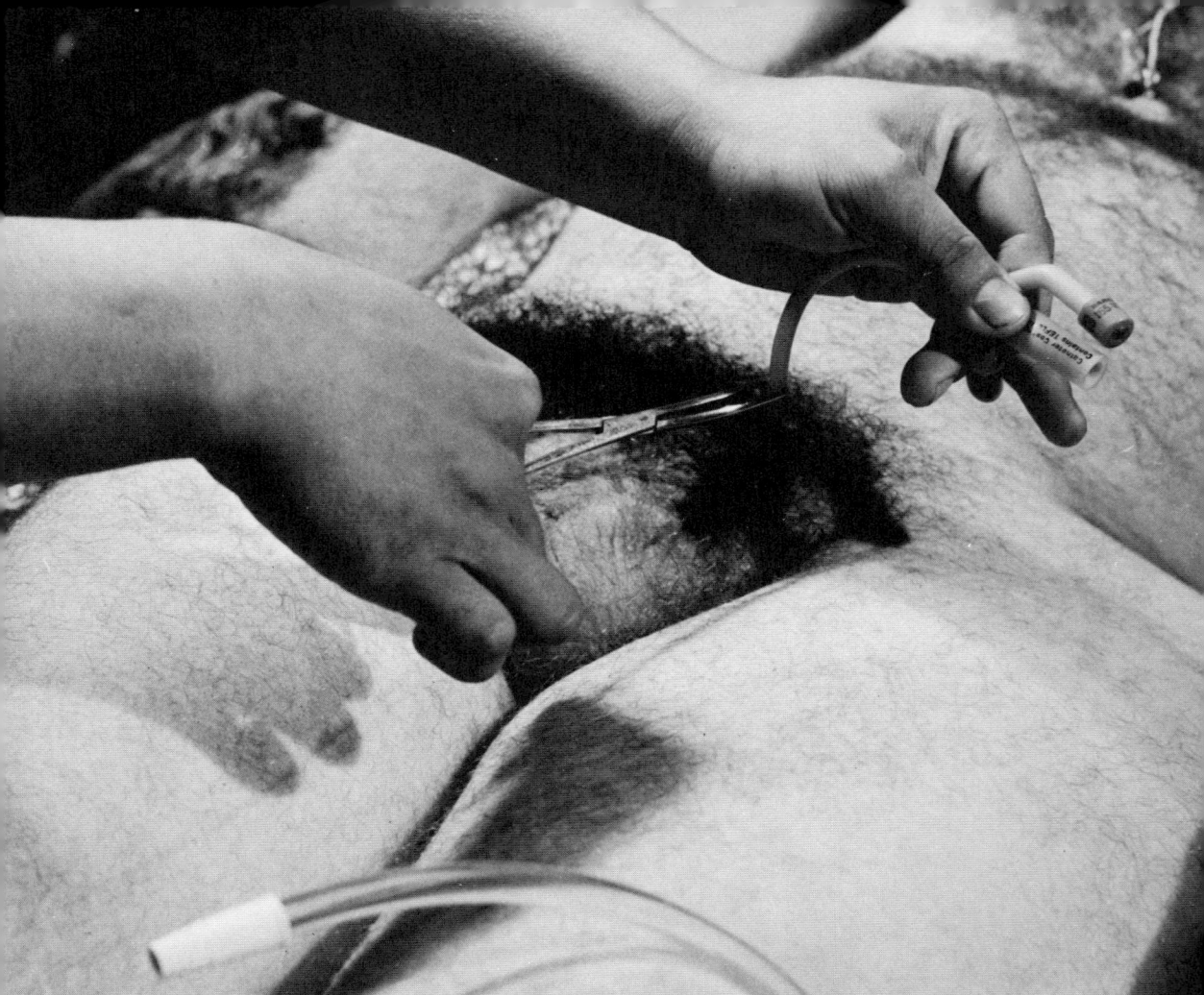

21

Because of the time you have spent in a medical facility and the attention that you have had to give to your body, you will be more knowledgeable than your partner about attaching your appliances, but you may have to ask your partner either to help you or even to do it alone. It is your responsibility to let him or her know what needs to be done.

There might be a few magic words after all — understanding, communication, imagination, experimentation — these can open up opportunities for a good relationship more quickly than you may think.

Whether you can manage alone or whether you need assistance while getting undressed, your partner may *want* to help you with your clothes or with the urine-collection bag that you may have strapped to your leg (22). When your partner is unable to assist you, a third person, such as an attendant, can help you get ready (23, 24).

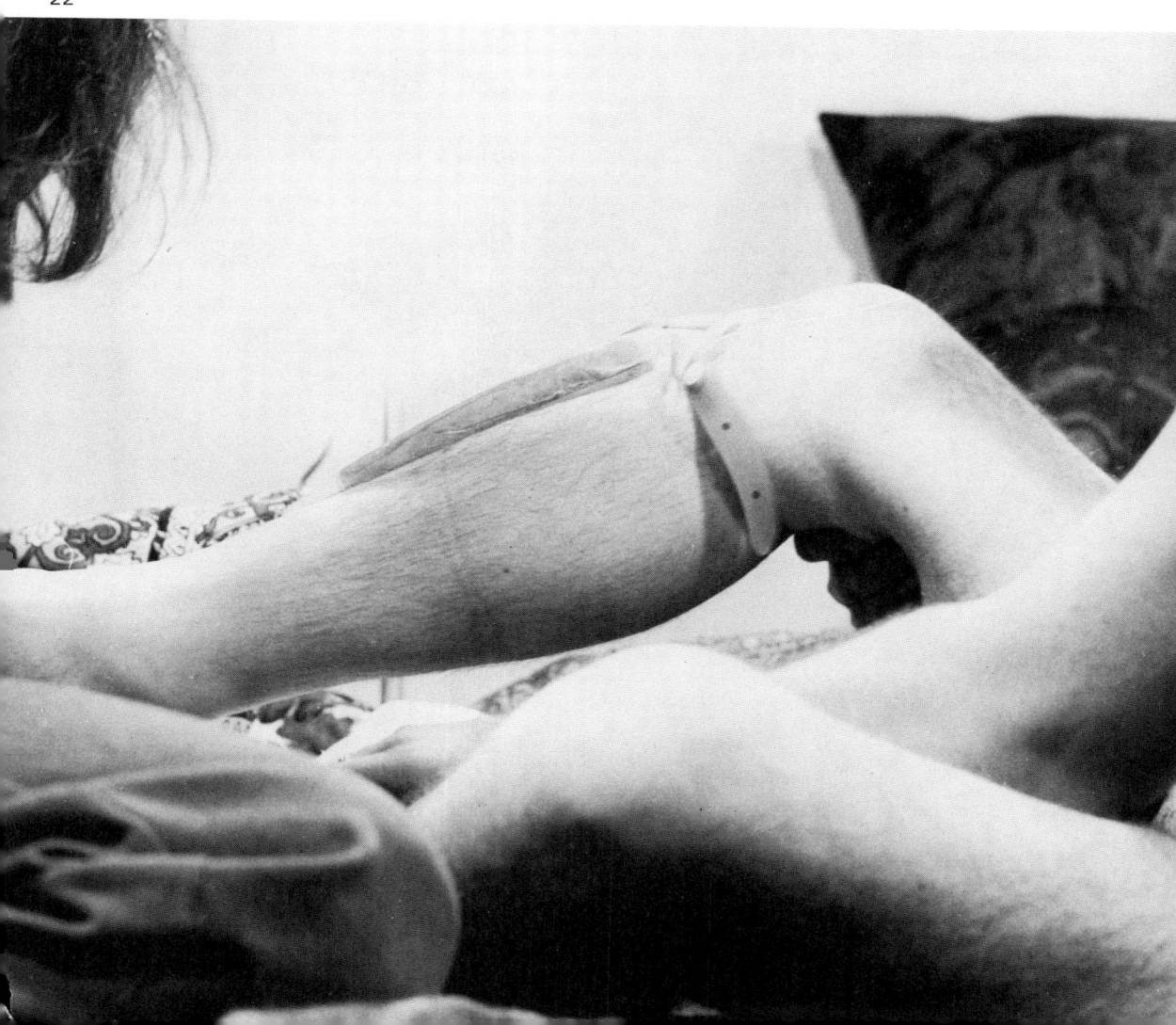

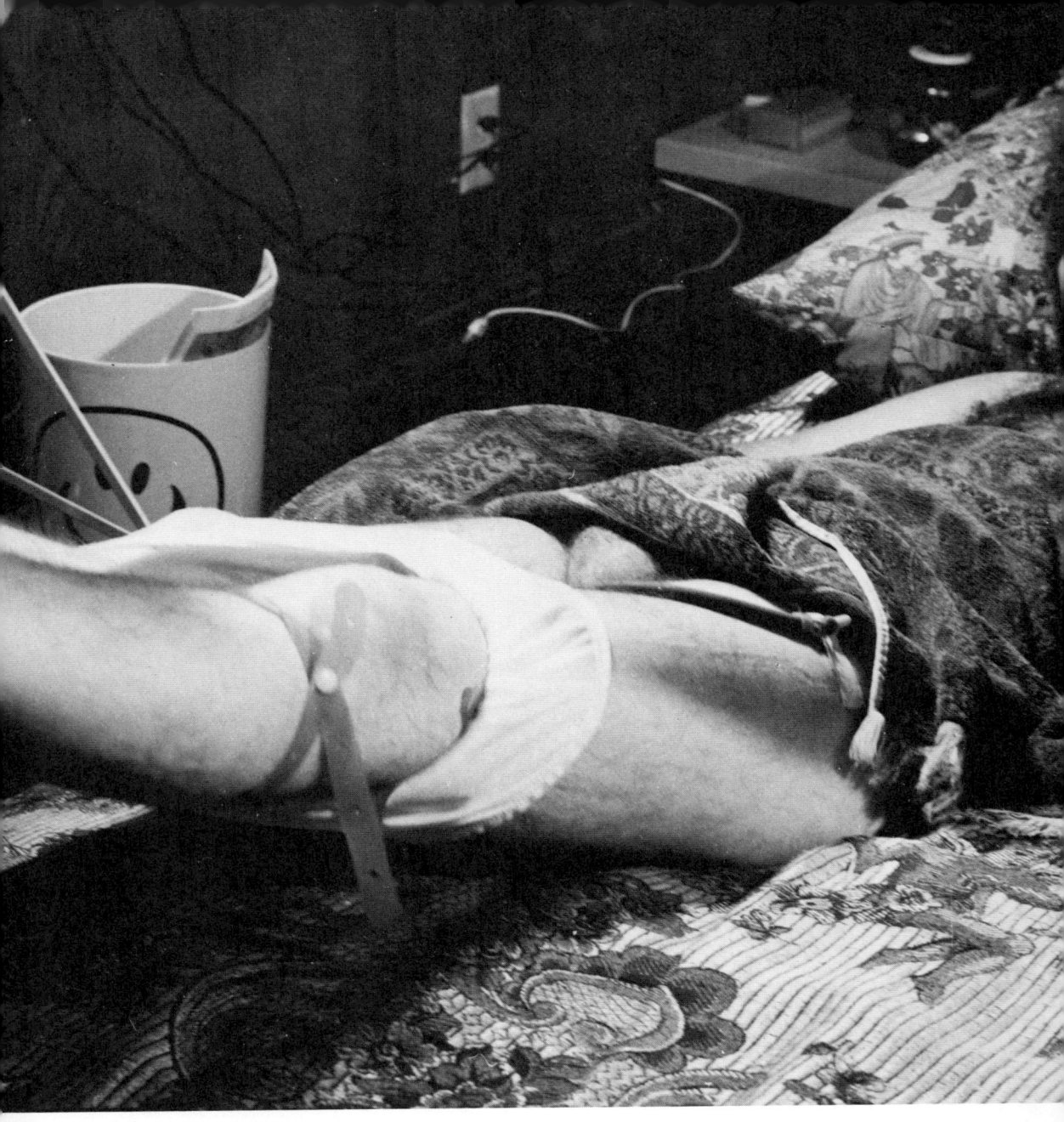

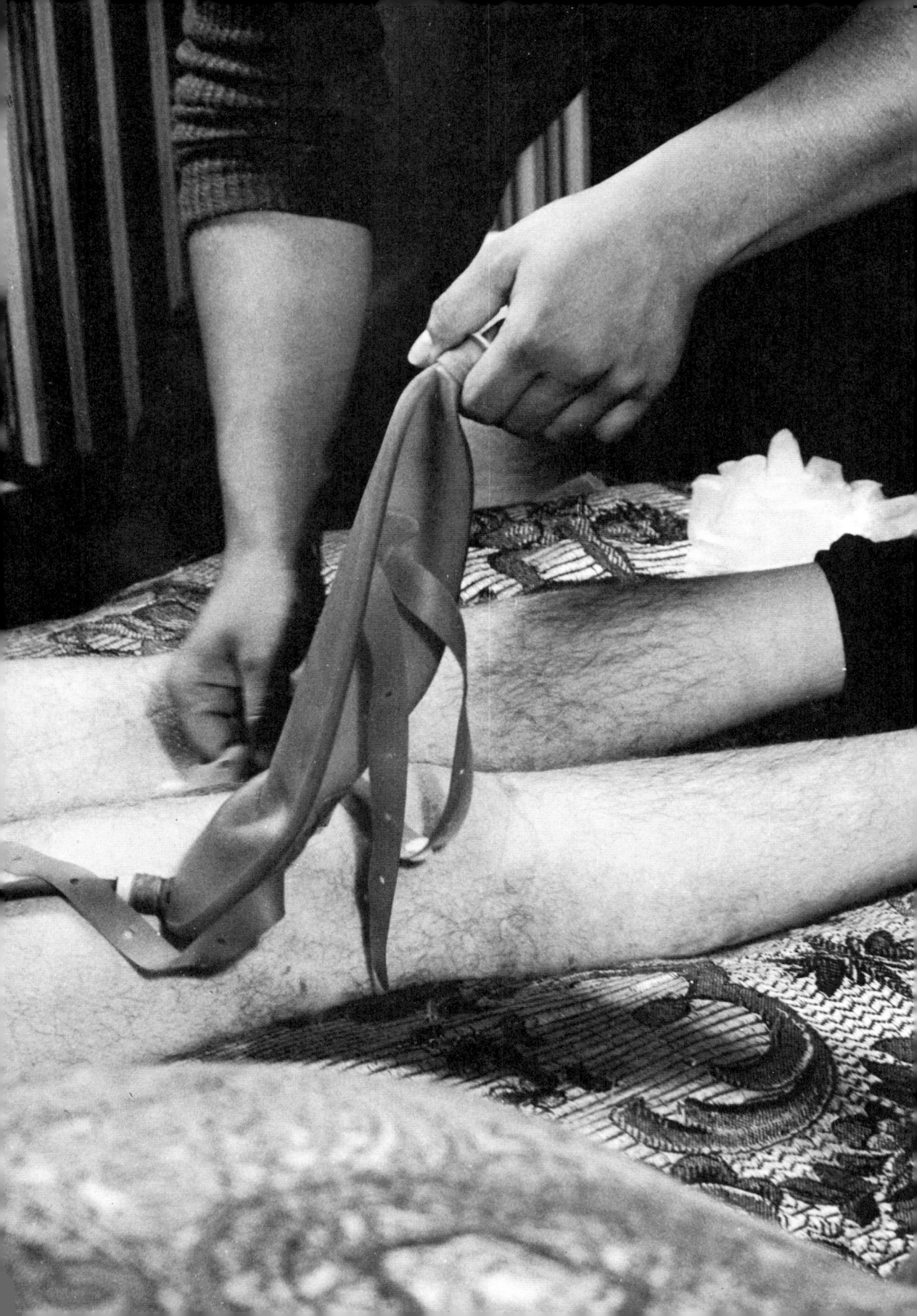

3 Arousal

There are an infinite number of turn-ons, and they are so much a part of a person's own sexual style that we only can tell you about some of the styles that others use to increase their enjoyment.

By talking to each other about sexual topics, fantasies, or the activities about to be experienced, the mere verbalization of the sensations or reactions can bring you and your partner to such a level of arousal that you both will be ready for physical contact. You can do these things while you are getting undressed, cleaning up, and getting into position. Talking together and touching one another in a tender, sensuous way while eating, drinking, or just being close to each other in a comfortable spot, is also fun. You can be kissing, hugging, petting, or caressing each other while listening to music or watching television, either on a couch or in your wheelchair, inside, outside, or in a car. When you have the inclination, any place where privacy will be assured is fine.

Experienced partners can position themselves to allow for pleasurable touching and feeling of one another (25). The able-bodied partner can more easily position his or her body in such a way as to allow sexual activity by the paraplegic or quadriplegic partner (26).

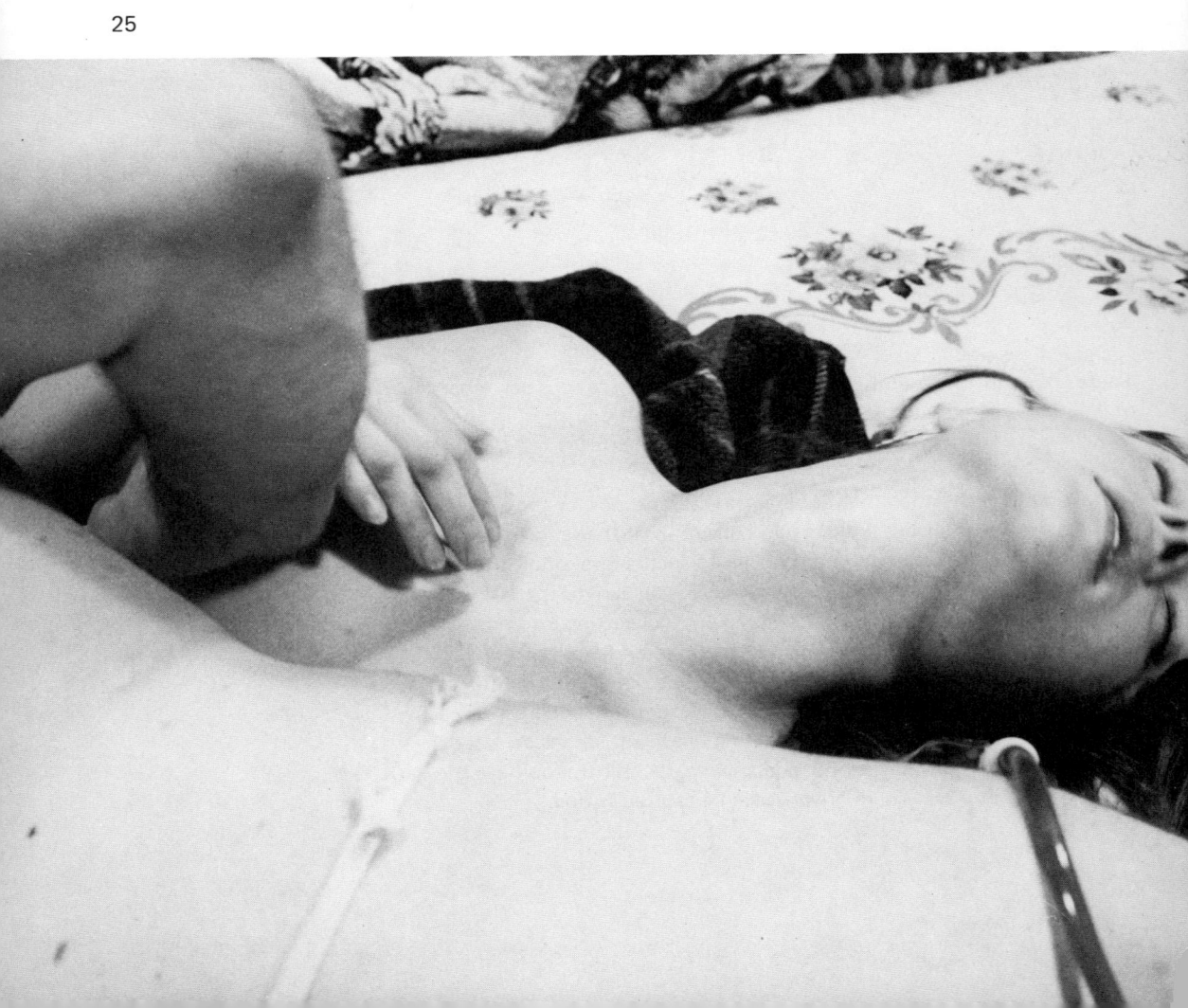

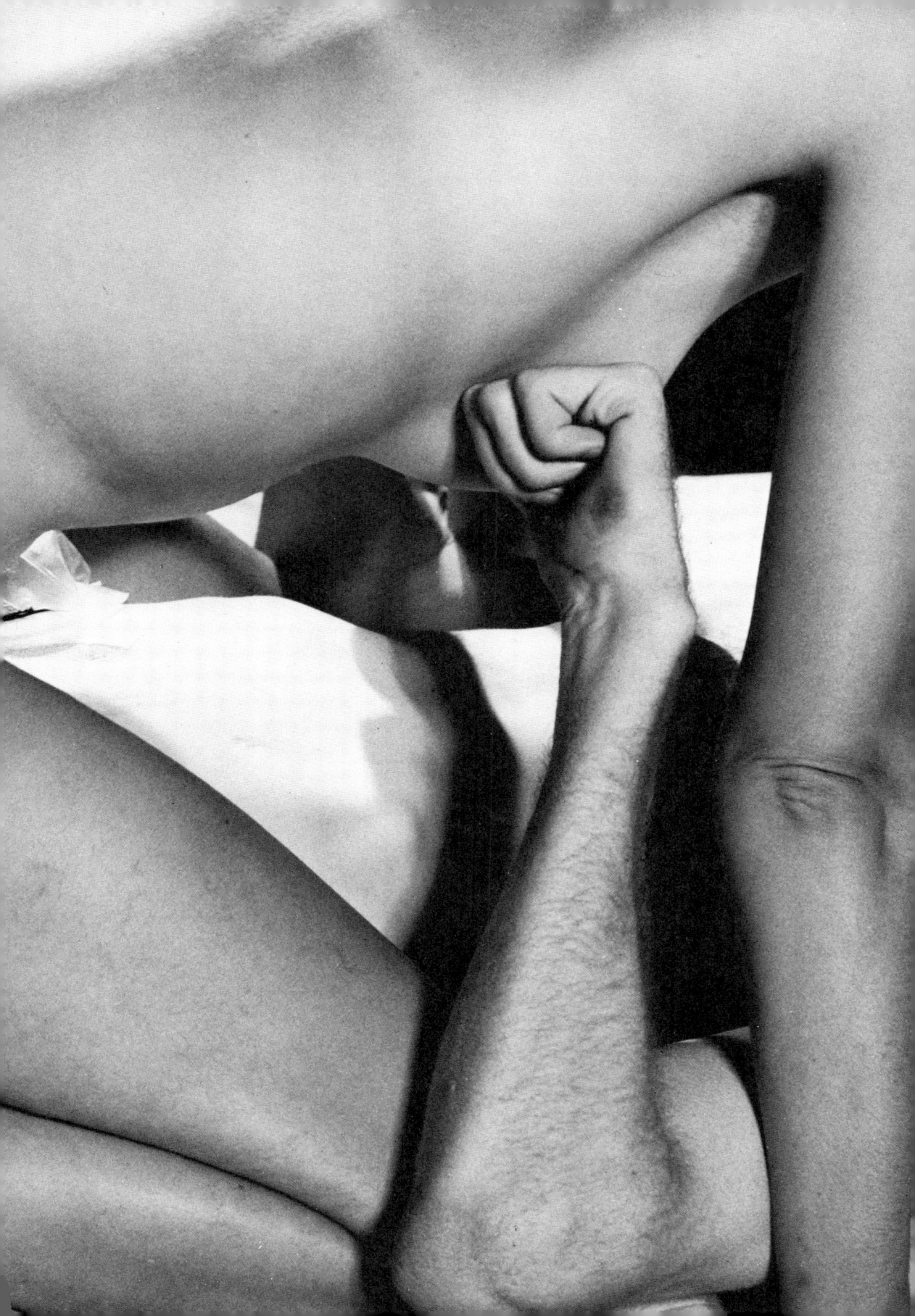

Whether you prefer to begin while resting on the floor, on a couch, or in a bed, you may find that stroking your partner's breasts, vagina, or penis, having your partner stroke yours, or both simultaneously, or giving each other a massage can be very stimulating for both of you. This can be done with your hands or with a vibrator, of which there are different types. A battery-powered vibrator, which can be used for a turn-on of either partner, is shown in photograph 27.

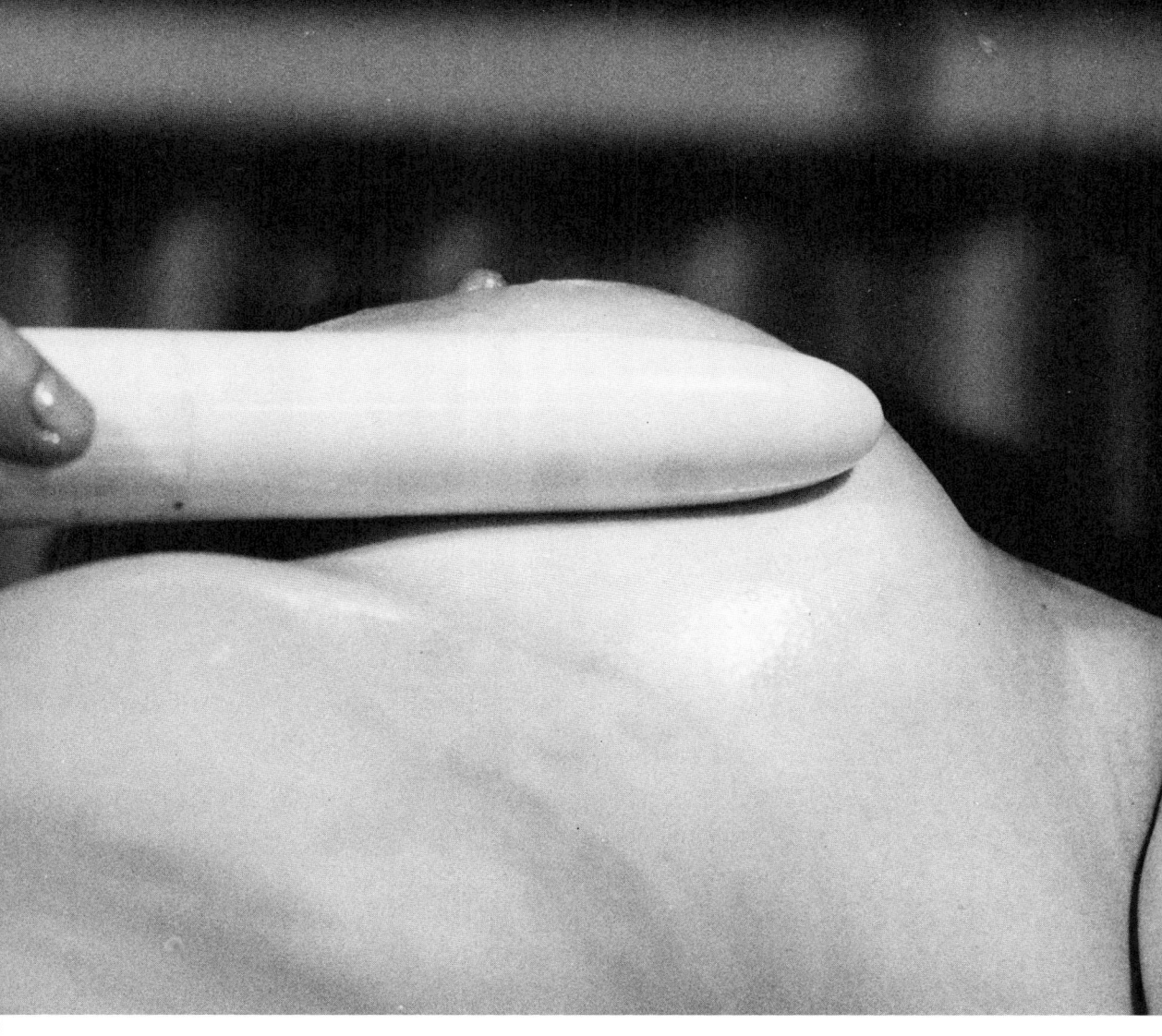

You do not necessarily need a lot of dexterity in your hands if you know where to touch or massage your partner. The breasts of some women, able-bodied and paraplegic, can sometimes be stimulated enough by her partner's mouth or hand to bring her close to, if not actually to, a climax; for some women it is like massaging or rubbing the area around the vagina. Male paraplegics sometimes have a heightened sensitivity in their breasts, and it can be exciting to them when the breasts are nibbled or rubbed. Body contact, sensations of skin on sensitive areas, the pressure of body weight, or gentle squeezing or fondling of your partner's genitals can be a tremendous turn-on for you and your partner (28, 29).

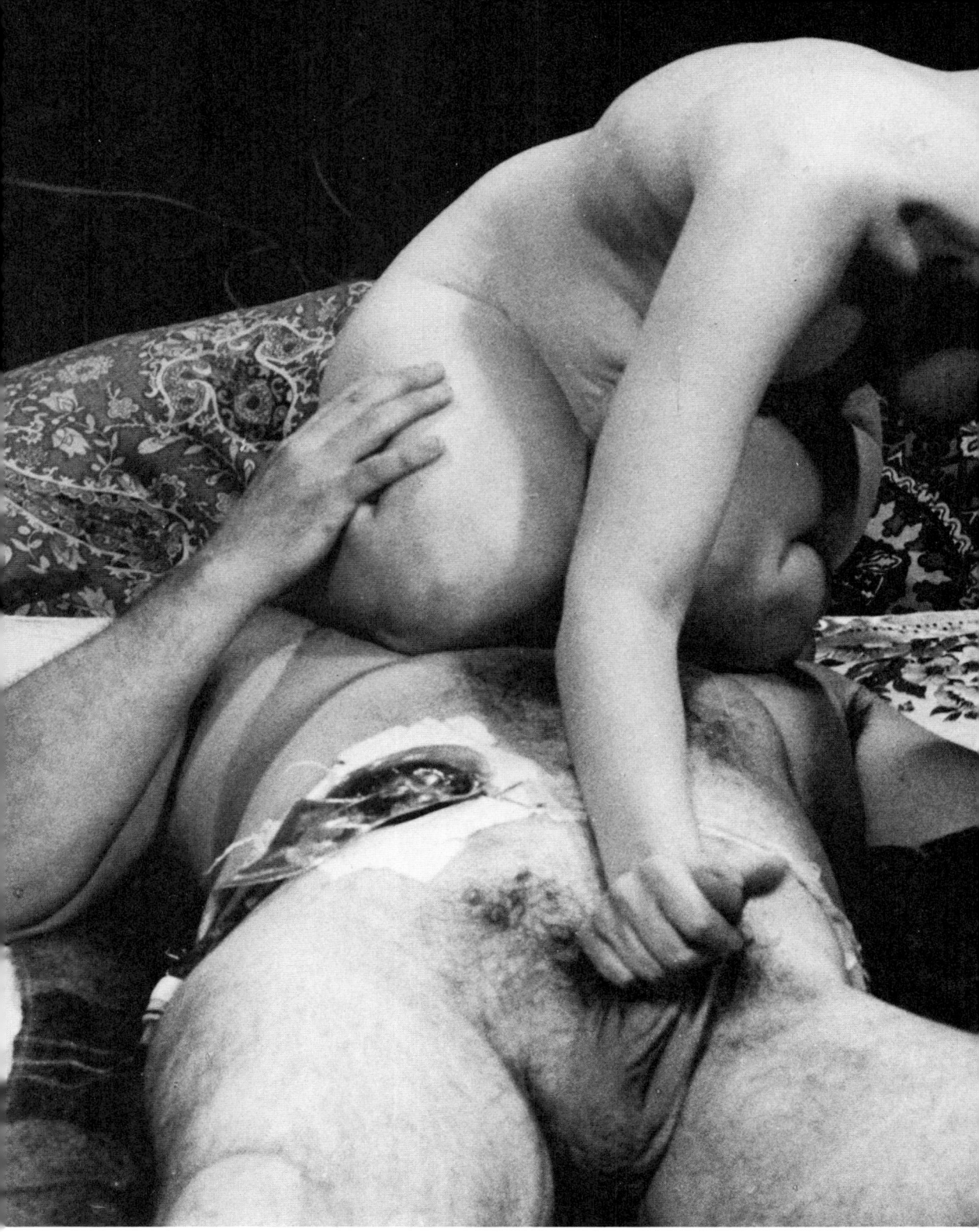

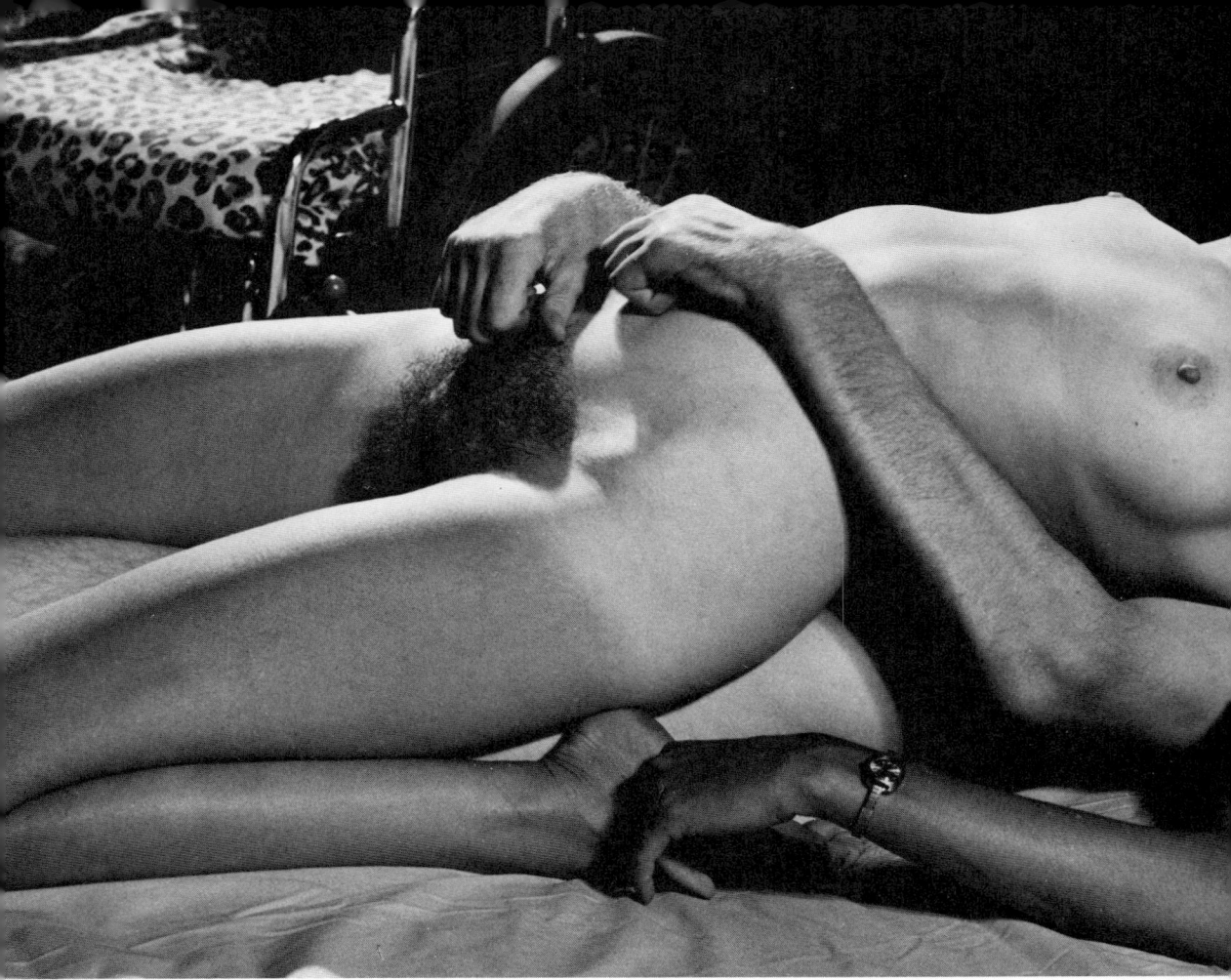

Not only is the pleasant smell and taste of love oils a turn-on, but if you and your partner choose to use the option of oral-genital stimulation or if you are just licking or sucking parts of each other, the oils enhance the sensations (30). There are many types of oils — some are scented and some are flavored. Not only do they give you a pleasant smell and taste sensation, but they also serve as a lubricant. Saliva also is a good lubricant, but it can dissipate faster than a cream or lotion. By ranging from K-Y Lubricating Jelly to coconut oil and Kama Sutra love oils, you can find that it is fun and exciting to experiment.

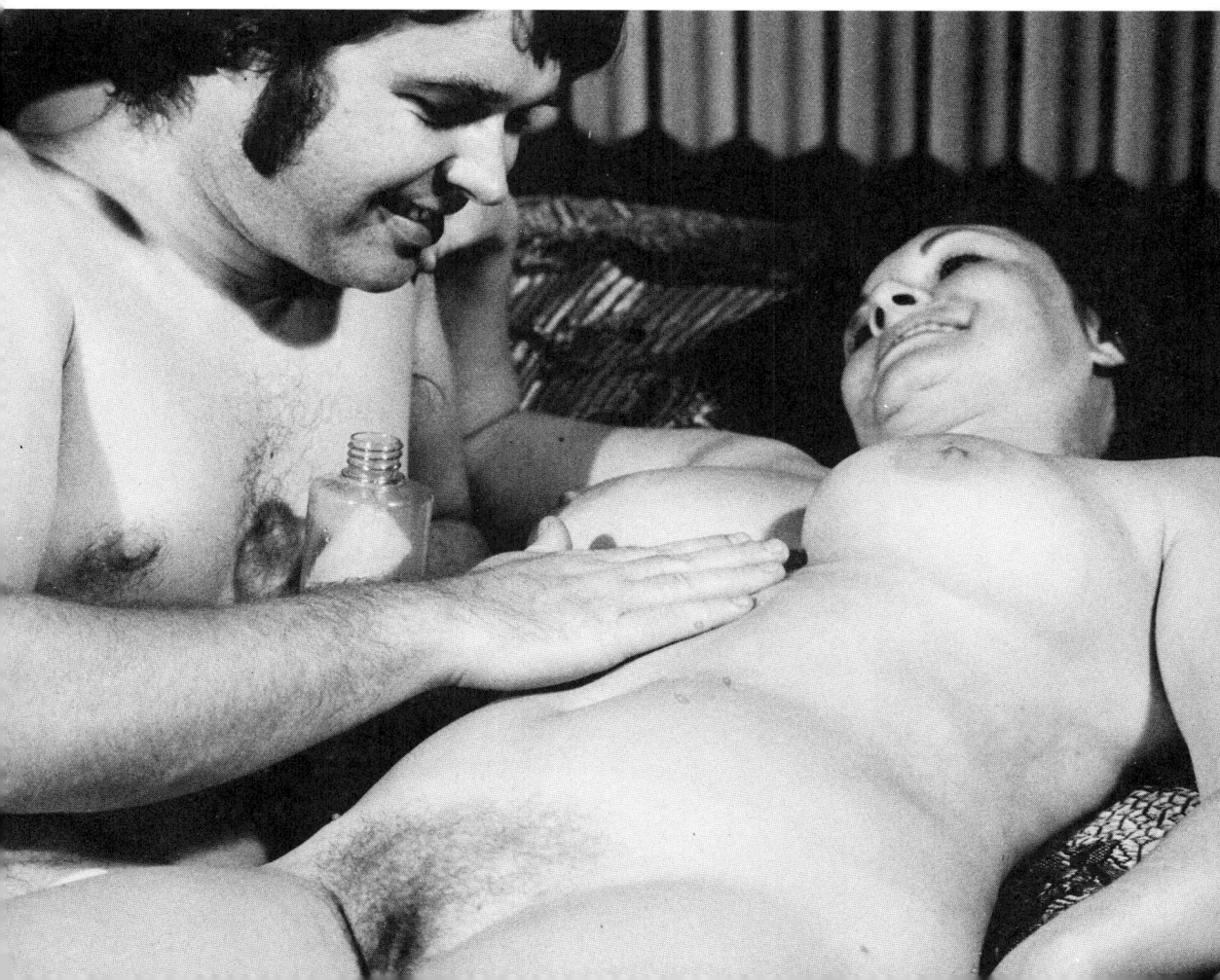

Using mirrors and having good lighting in the room enables you to view each other's reactions better. Electric or battery-powered vibrators are especially nice for massaging if your hands lack dexterity (31). Candles, incense, reading, poetry, music — the possibilities are endless. If there is one rule to follow, it is to use your imagination and experiment with anything you can think of as long as your partner is willing. Finding out what turns each other on is fun and can be enjoyable and rewarding to both of you.

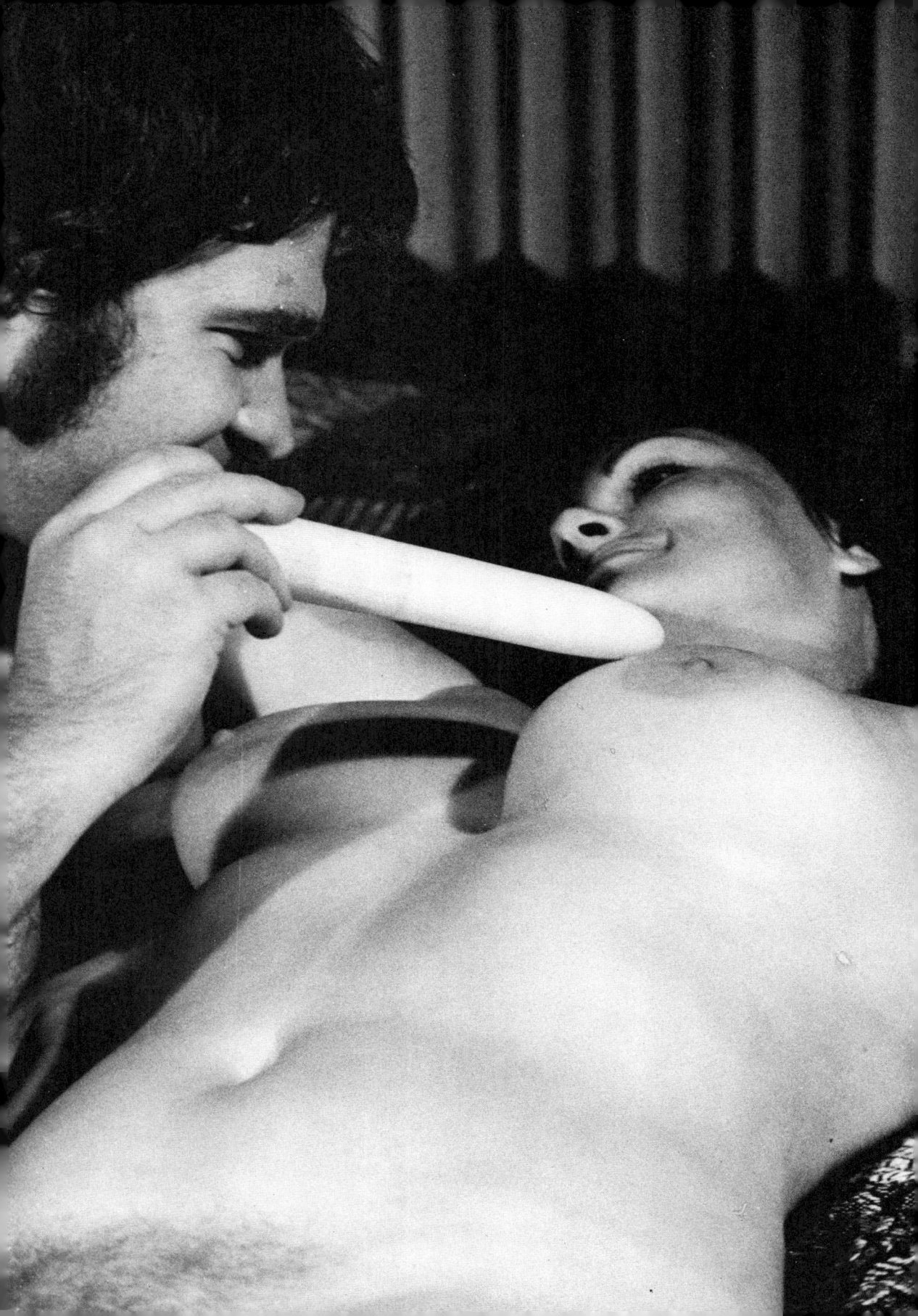

A reflex erection of the penis results from internal or external stimulation around the penis. Often, it can be achieved by manipulation with the partner's hand (32) or any other technique that the couple finds satisfactory. This means that you, as a male paraplegic or quadriplegic, may be able to develop an erection sufficient for penetration and intercourse. The erection is similar to the reflex you can get from tapping your leg below the kneecap. Chemical or physical changes that you cannot feel or sense can sometimes bring on an erection.

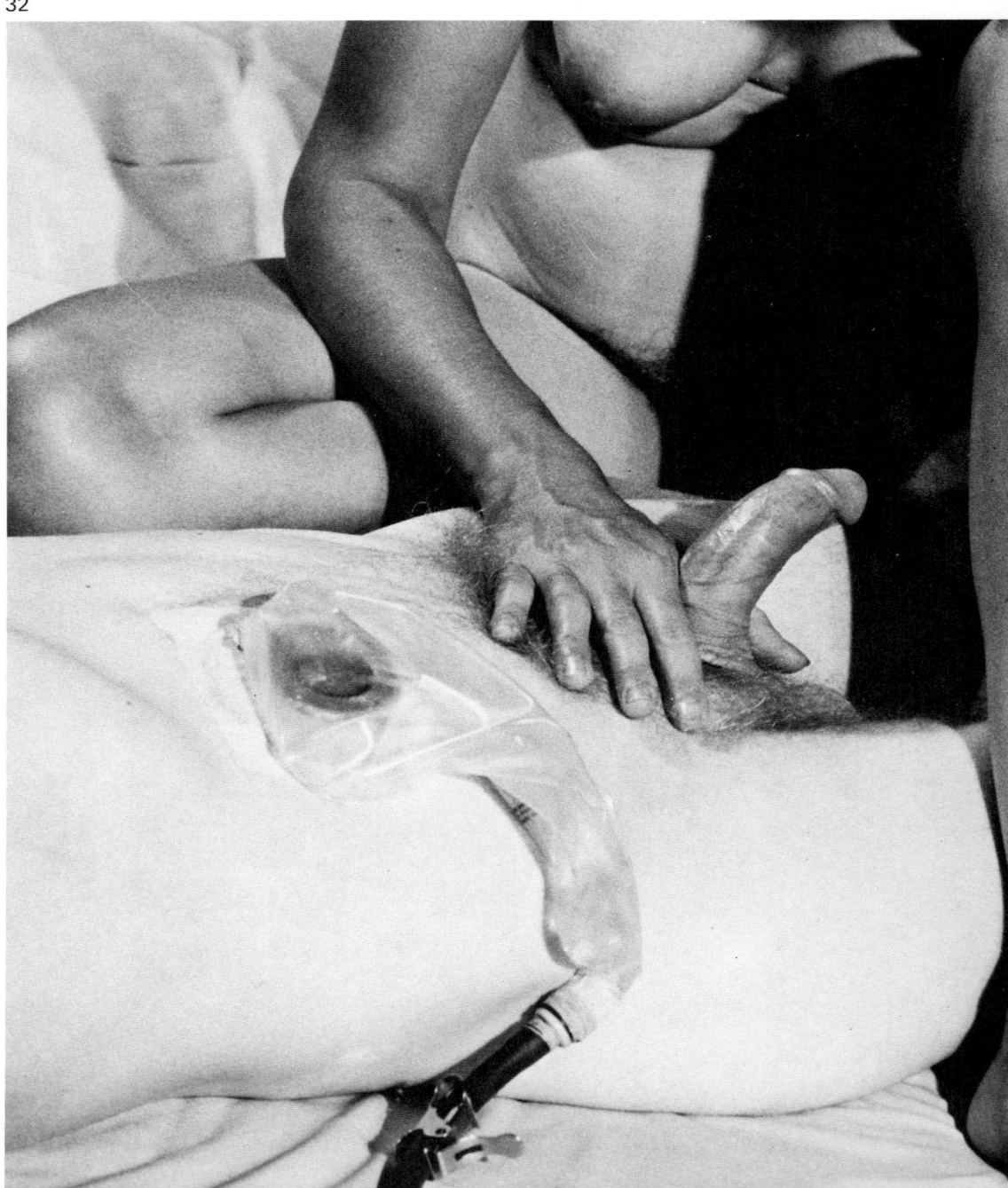

The most common cause of the erection is some type of stimulation of the penis or genital area. The types of stimulation that bring about an erection differ greatly from person to person, so you will have to find the right patterns of pressure and rhythm that work well for you. Having the room temperature chilly or cold may help one person achieve an erection but have no effect on another. Some say that irritation on the testicular sac, or scrotum, will cause an erection (33).

33

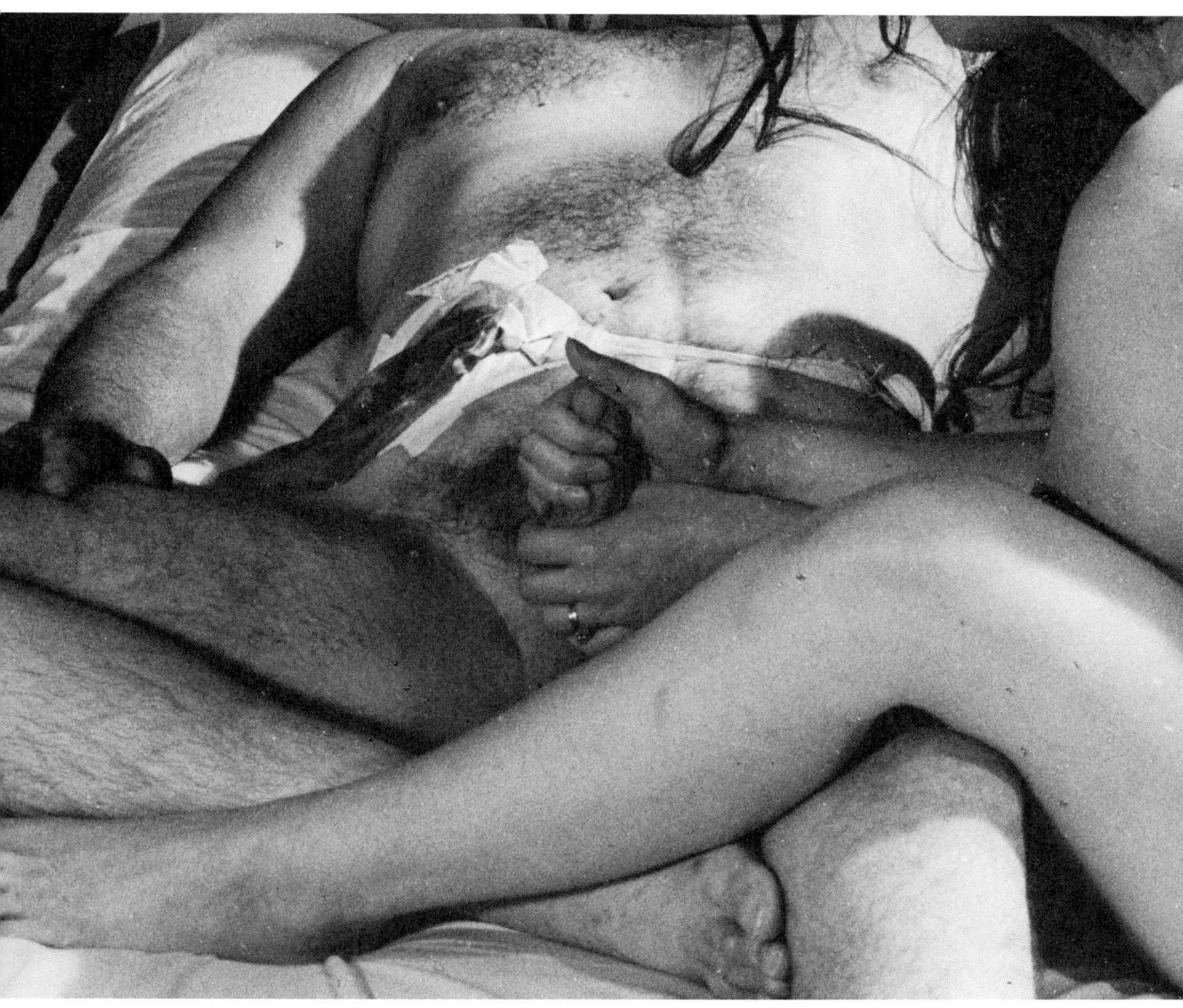

For some people, stimulation around the rectal opening helps to achieve an erection. If you have noticed yourself having an erection during, before, or after bowel emptying, you could possibly take advantage of that knowledge for purposes of your sex life.

In most cases the erection can be maintained for as long as stimulation is present. Continuing the same patterns of rhythm and pressure of the stimulation is important, for if the stimulation is changed drastically, the erection may be lost. Some say that a change in body position or movement does not affect their ability to maintain an erection. Others say that spasm or any change in their position and movements will not only result in a loss of the erection but will also cause them to urinate. However, only those who do not use catheters during sexual activity and those who remove them need to be concerned about the possibility of the bladder emptying. You will have to find out for yourself how physically passive or active you can be before you lose an erection. Again, the key is experimentation.

Stroking yourself, or masturbating by yourself or with your partner, to find out your own body responses, and trying out new and different techniques not only is fun and enjoyable, but will teach you a lot about your capabilities (34). Each person will learn the type of stimulation that works best for him. Sometimes, stimulation must be gentle and rhythmical and at other times vigorous in order to achieve an erection (35, 36).

34

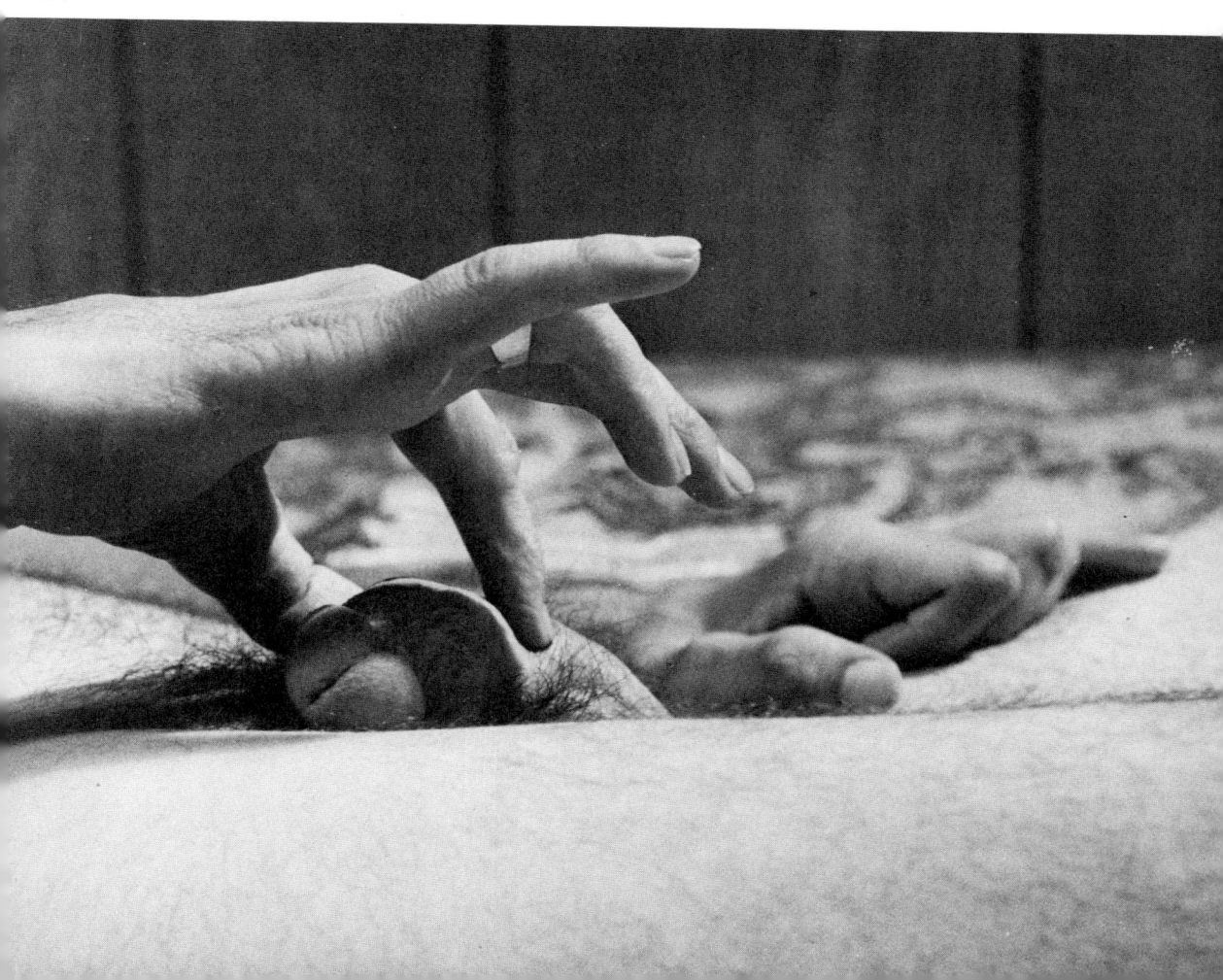

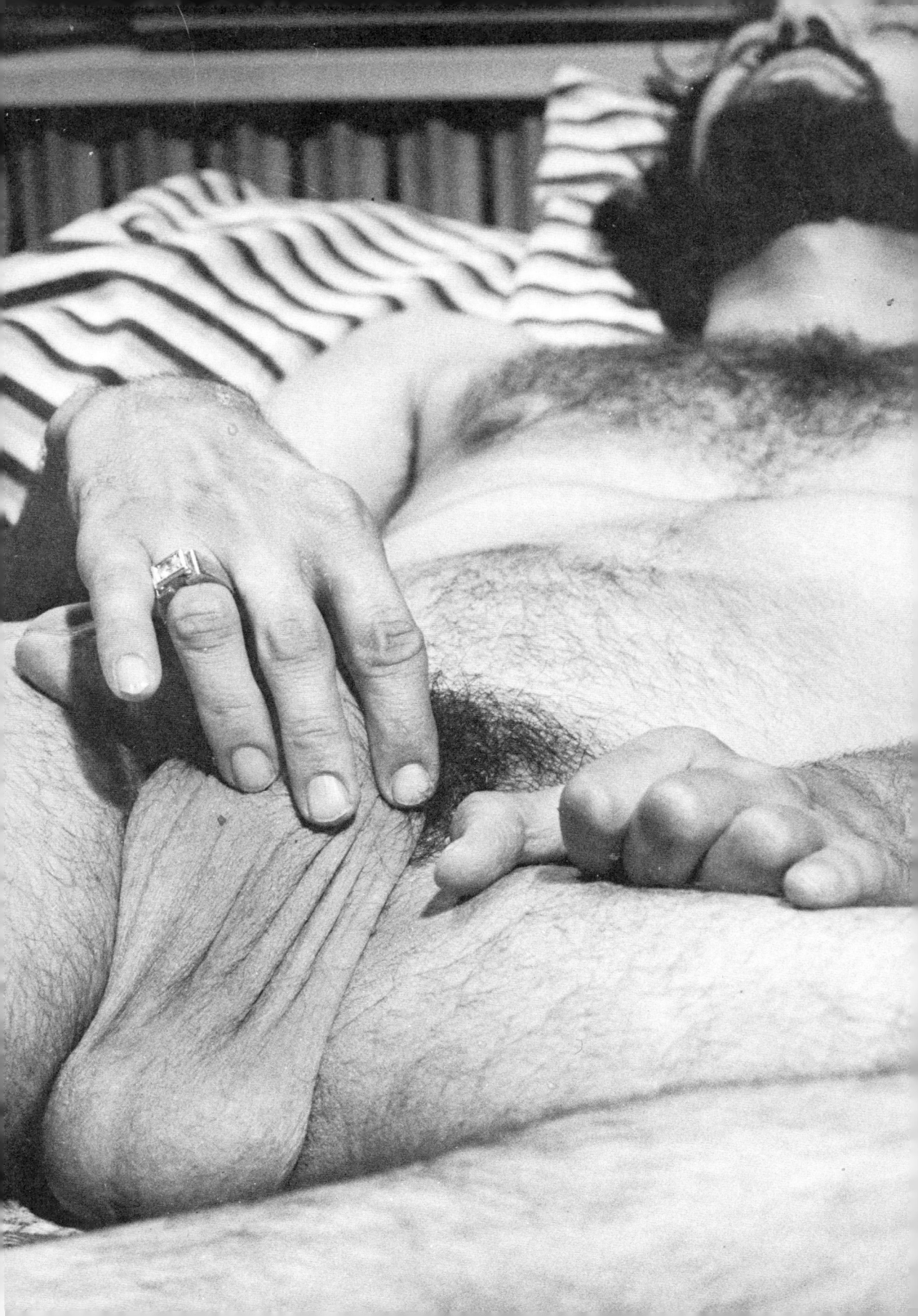

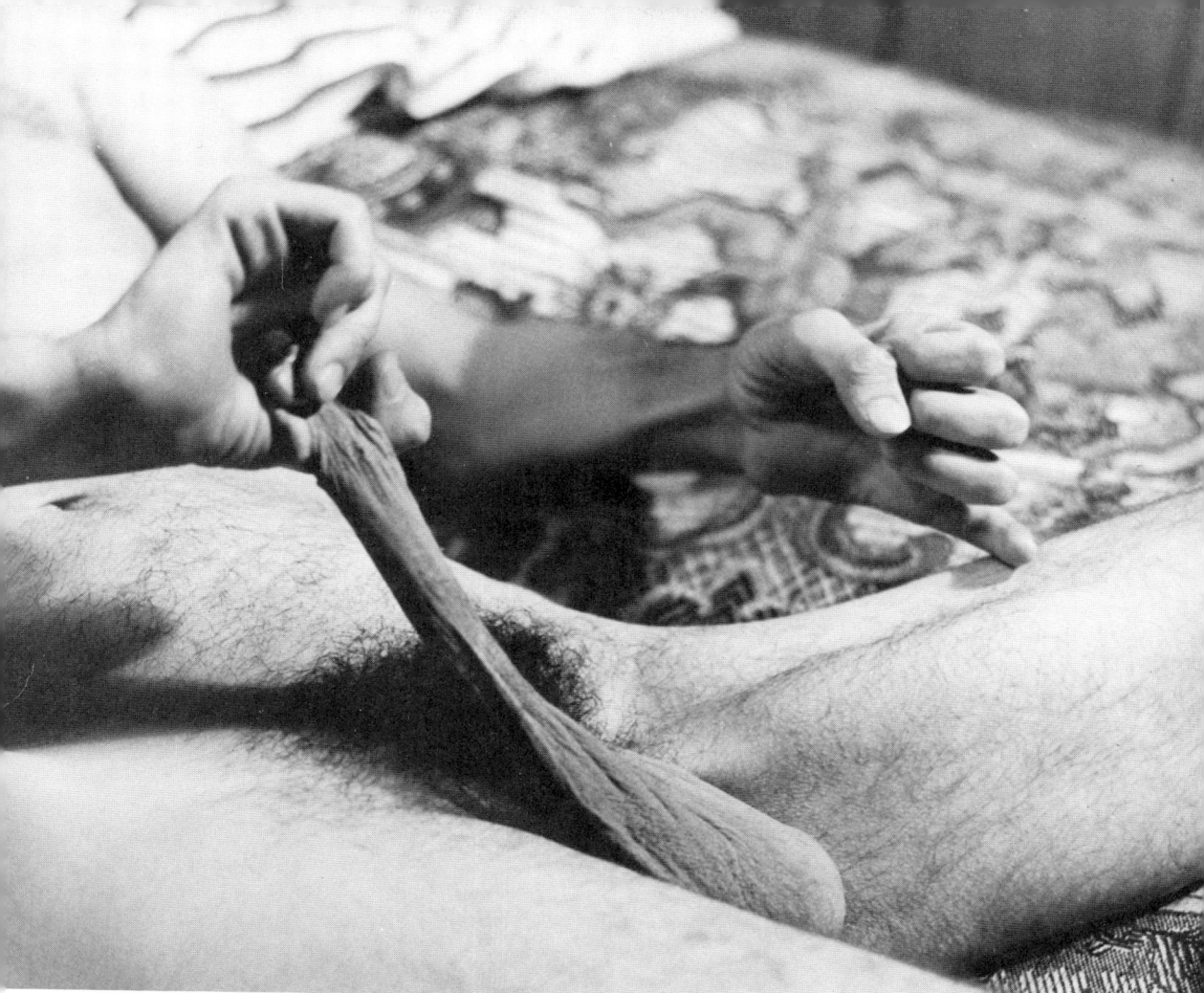

At times a reflex erection may not last or stay hard enough for penetration, so it is important to keep in mind that although an erection is desirable, it is not the only way to bring satisfaction to you and your partner. You also have hands, a mouth, a tongue and other body parts to use for this purpose. There is no area of the body that cannot be used for sexual expression, and the ways to use these areas for your partner's and your own enjoyment and satisfaction are numerous.

4 Intercourse

Men who have spinal cord injuries very low in the back may be unable to have a reflex erection at any time. In this situation a technique called *stuffing* could be especially helpful for you. This method can give your partner the sensation of holding the penis in the vagina without the need of an erection. In the stuffing technique, the disabled man can assume the dominant position and, with his fingers, tuck his flaccid, soft penis into the vagina (37–42). By thrusting her hips and using the muscles of the vagina, his partner takes the soft penis into her vagina with a sort of pulling, sucking movement. While the flaccid penis gives a sensation of penetration that can be very satisfying in itself, the motion of the hips and the muscle action of the vagina often cause a reflex erection in men who are unable to have one. The Kegel exercises (see the Glossary) can aid the able-bodied woman in developing these muscles to a high degree, which can also heighten her enjoyment. The stuffing technique may also be used by a male with a high-level injury. His able-bodied partner can kneel over him and use her fingers for tucking the penis into her vagina; she can also tighten her vaginal muscles and use the pelvic movements mentioned previously.

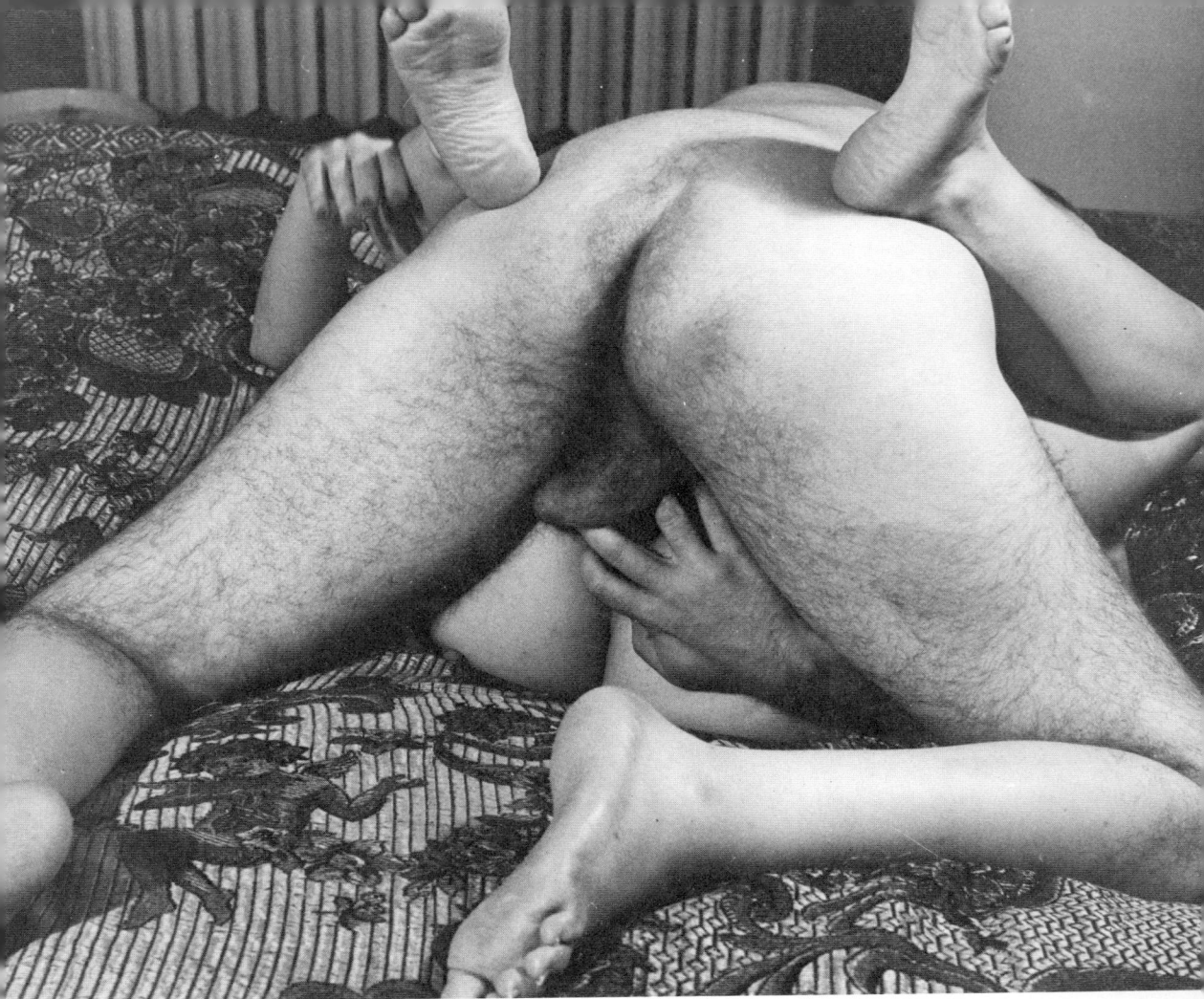

38

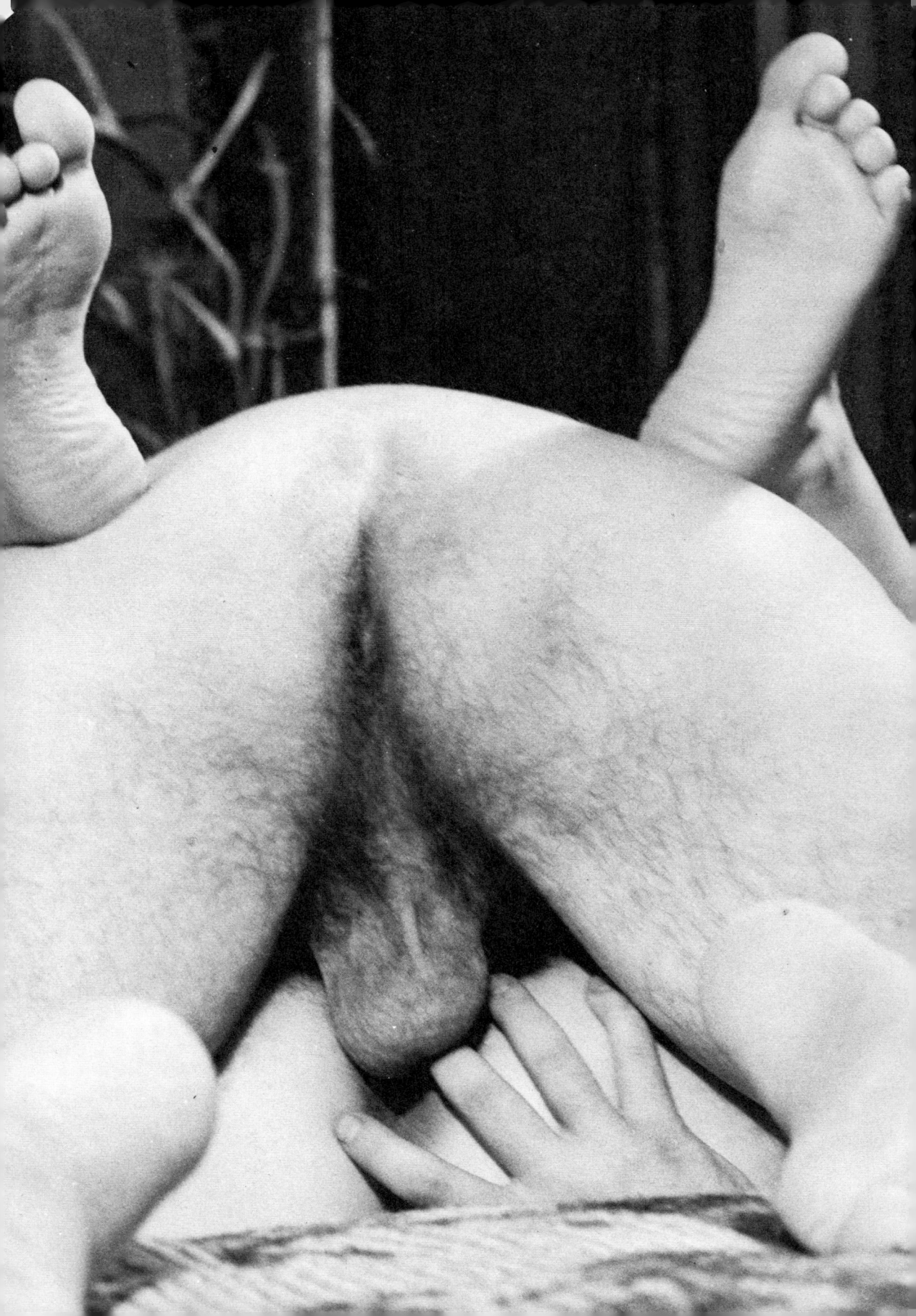

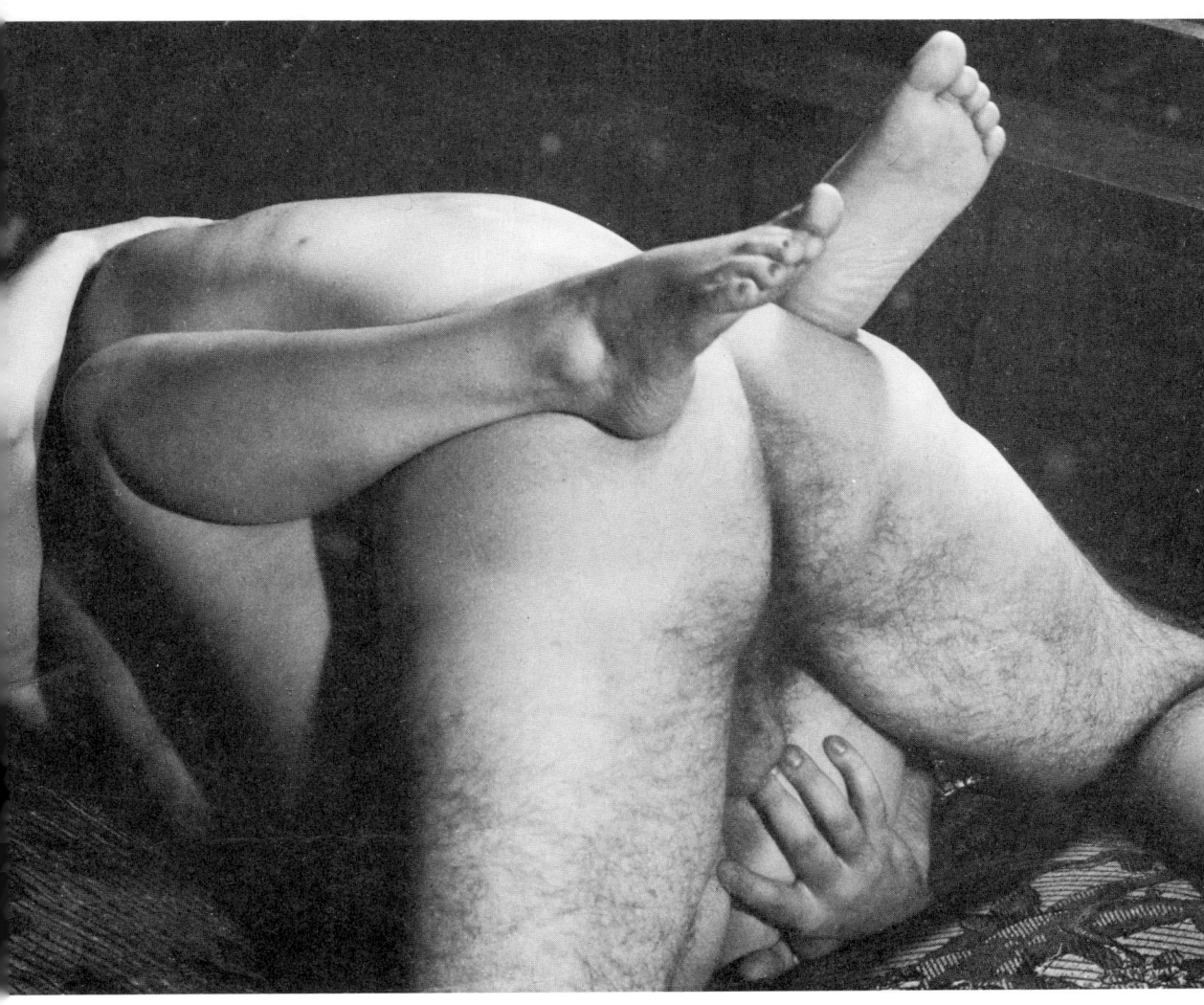

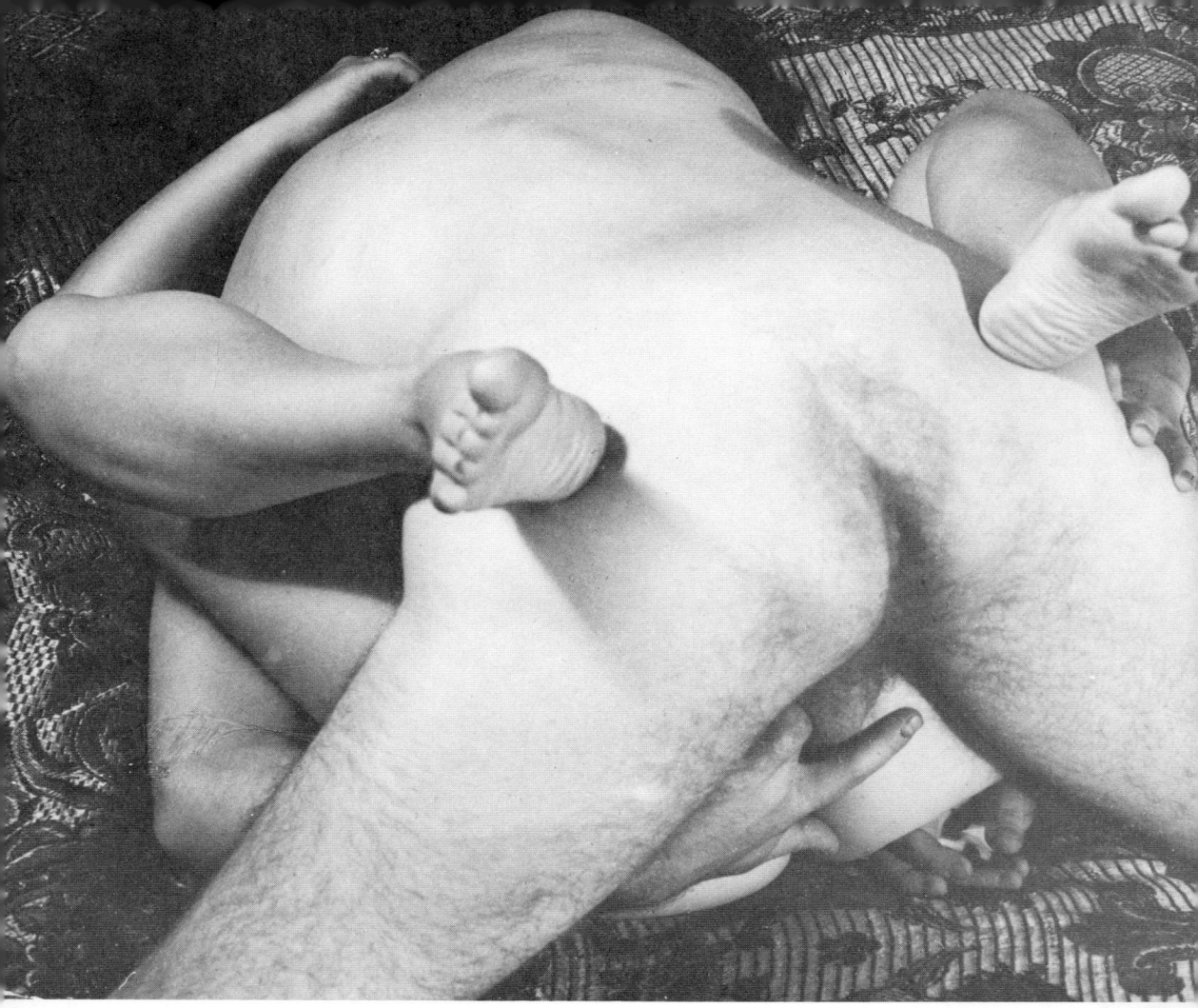

41

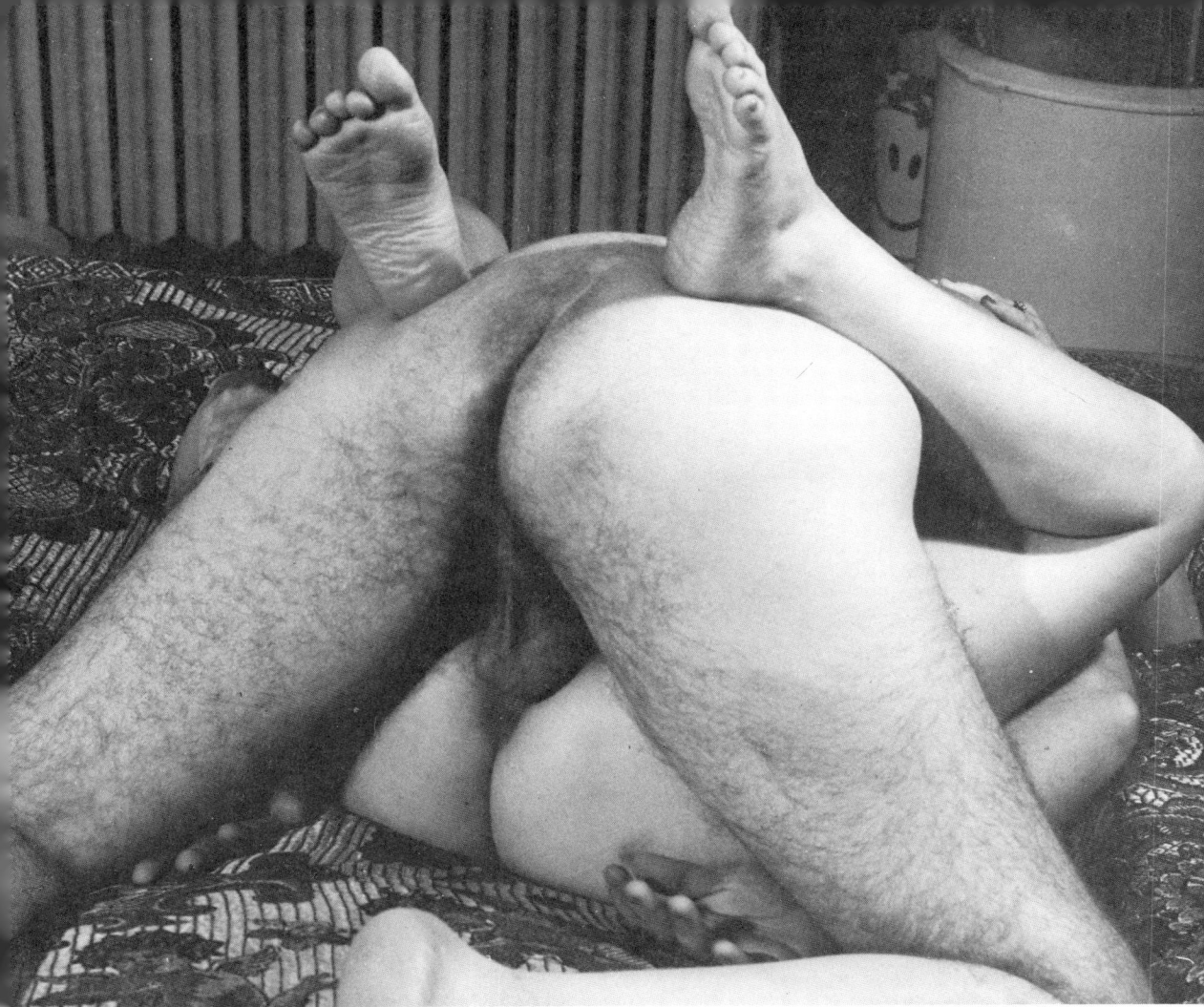

Whether you are a male or female paraplegic or quadriplegic, the positions that are possible for intercourse are limited only to your individual abilities and inclinations. Your disability will, of course, have an influence on the positions and methods that you will be able to use. Many of the positions that will be described have different advantages that could apply to your own situation. You will find that some are better for achieving motion for the active stroking and thrusting of intercourse, while others will seem to be more passive. Success will depend on what you find works well for you. We hope that the following description of techniques will give you some ideas to try.

If you are a female paraplegic or quadriplegic and your partner assumes the position on top, your legs can be placed around him. Your legs can also be held up to your chest so that your partner is lying on the back side of your thighs. In this position he can achieve good penetration, but it can limit your movements. You can use your hands and arms for some thrusting movement or, by using your hands to push your buttocks together, give your partner the feeling of a vaginal squeeze and more pressure on his penis. You can also use your arms on another part of his body to give him and you more pleasure.

If you are a paraplegic male, with practice you can learn to have intercourse in the on-top position. If your arms are strong, you can achieve a great deal of friction and motion between the penis and vagina by doing push-ups from the on-top position (43). You can balance on your arms or move a little off to one side of your partner and use an elbow or shoulder for support, or combine these movements. Positioning your knees by bending them and spreading them apart a little, gives your partner the room for hip movement and upward thrust; or you may be able to achieve a downward thrusting motion by rocking or shifting your weight back and forth. Your partner may be able to support most of your weight and enable you to supply most of the movements by bringing her knees up to her chest and having you lie on her legs and knees. Her feet will then be alongside your hips and can keep you from sliding off to one side and out of position. You will then have the opportunity to rock back and forth, supplying most of the movement with your arms and your knees, which you are using for support and balance. You should try as much as possible to keep your weight off of your partner's buttocks and pelvic area to allow her the opportunity for movement.

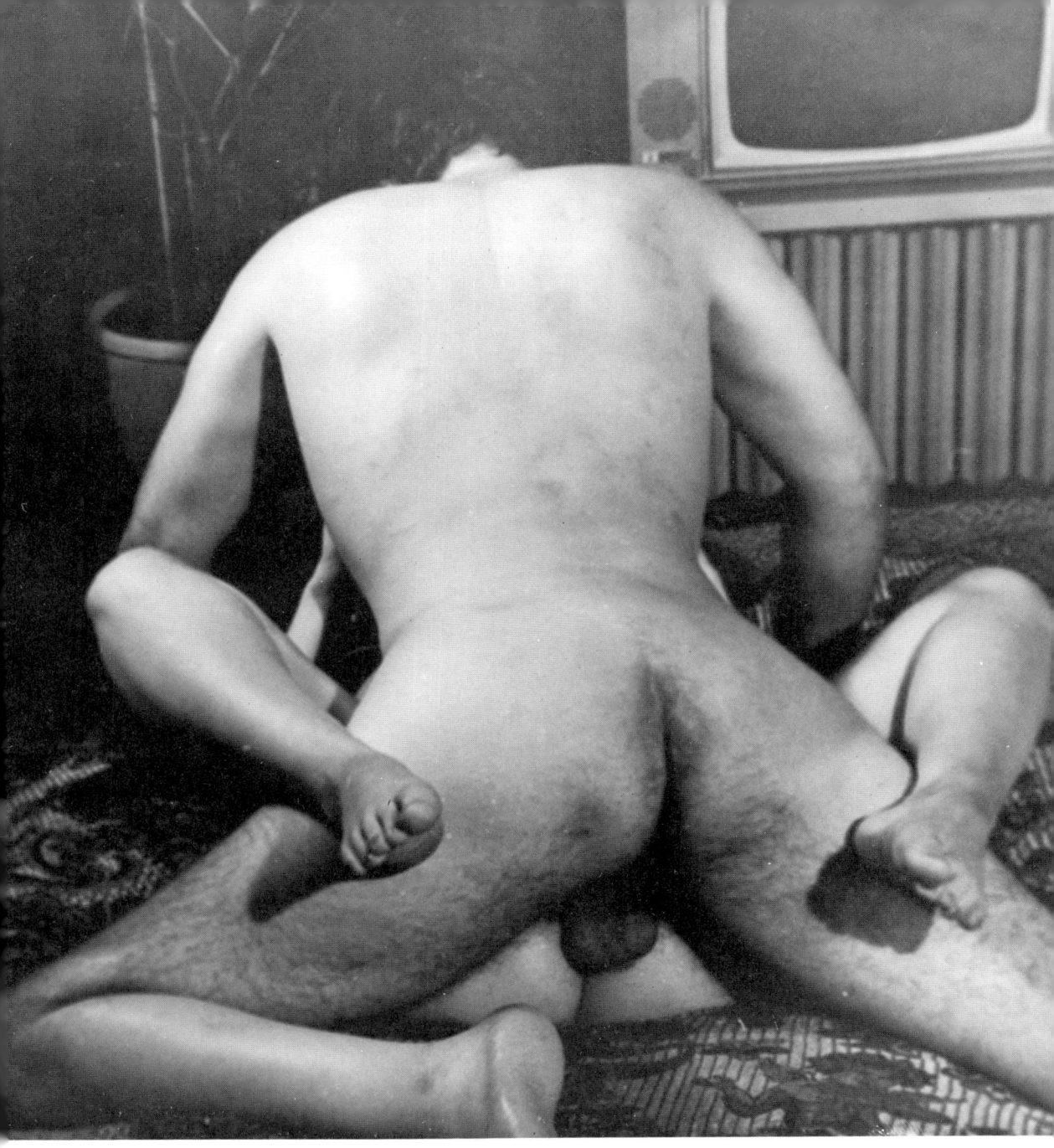

When the woman assumes the position on top of you, the disabled male partner (44—46), and has her legs straddling your body, she will then have more freedom for hip and pelvic movement; also, by not having to support your weight, she may be more comfortable. You will then have both hands free to help with her body rhythm or to rub or stroke another part of her body. If you are the disabled female, you can straddle your partner's body and, by using your hands and arms around his neck or shoulders, pull yourself up and down and achieve a pelvic lifting motion. This way you can supply most or all of the movement. Your partner's hands will then be free either to help your rhythm or balance or to caress another part of you to increase the enjoyment for both of you.

44

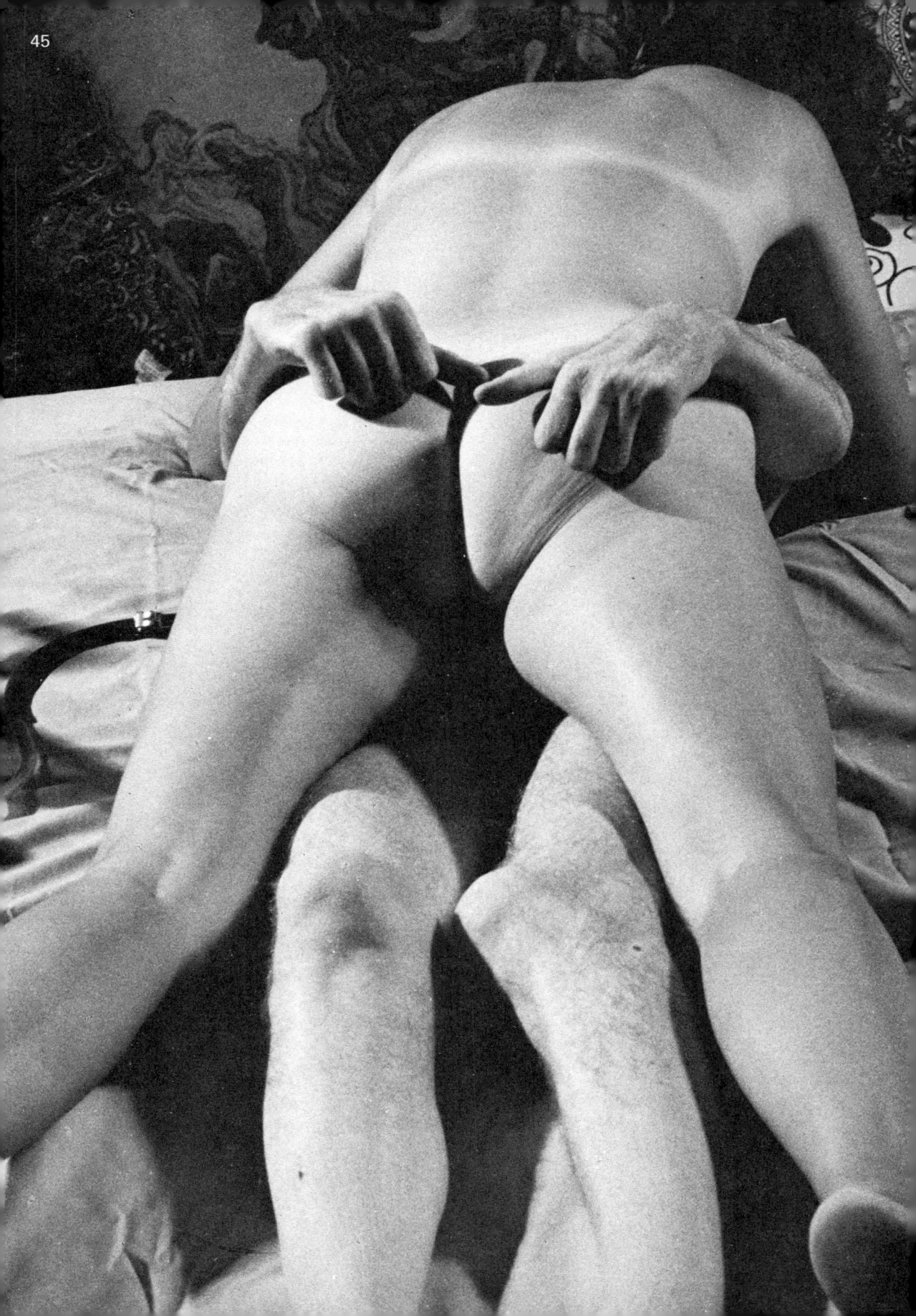

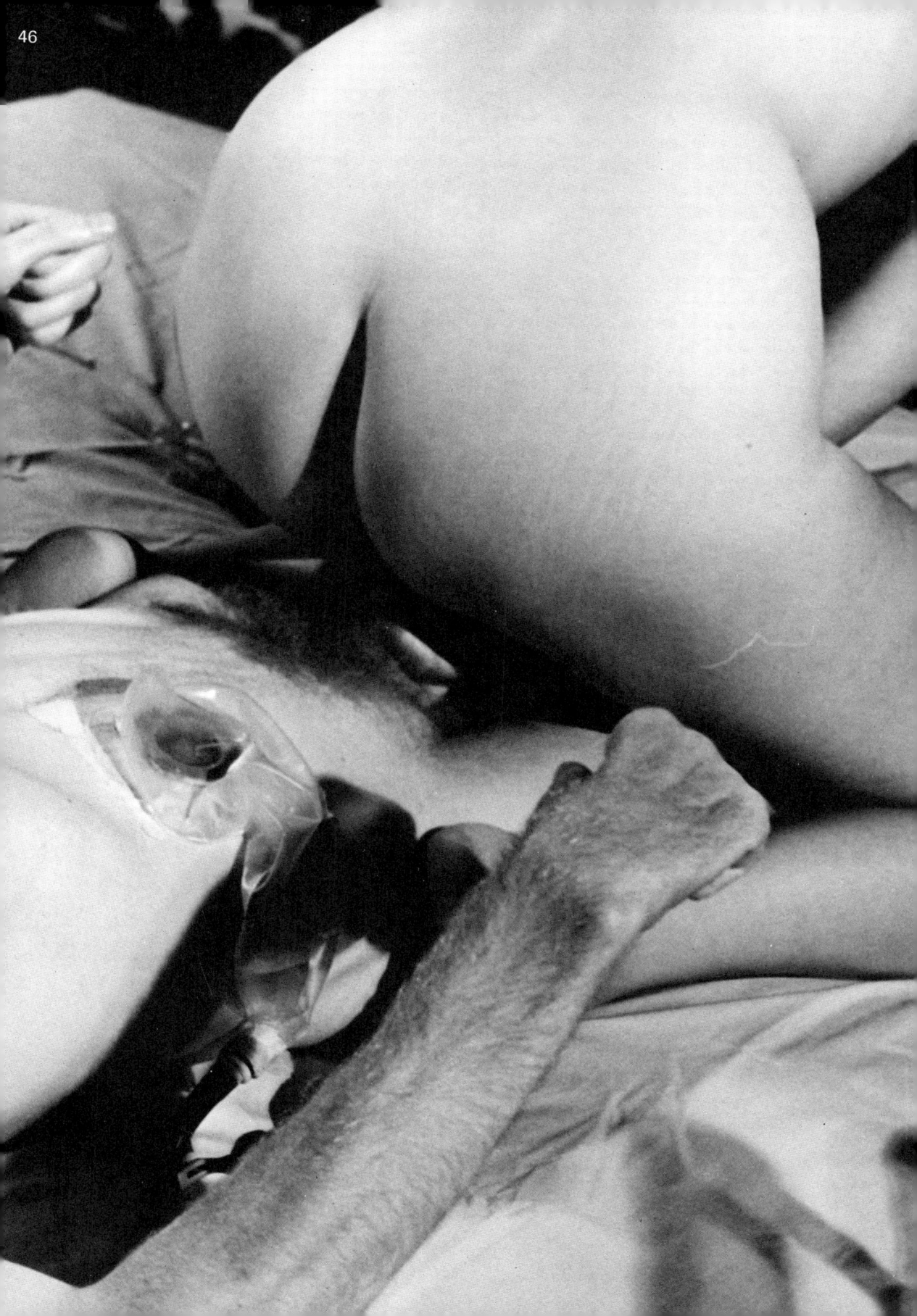

This position can easily be varied to a sitting position. The woman puts her legs around her partner, keeping them slightly bent and letting her buttocks slide between his legs as both sit up holding their arms around each other to help support each other's weight and to keep from falling backward. The penis will maintain penetration, and although the motion of the woman's hips is slowed, the closeness to each other can make up for the loss of movement.

Sitting in and using the wheelchair for intercourse can be fun, but you may run into many gymnastic and positioning difficulties. If you are a disabled male and are face-to-face with the woman straddling you in the wheelchair, she will have the problem of where to put her legs to avoid the wheels and arms of the wheelchair getting in the way. Penetration of the vagina from the rear, with the woman sitting with her back to you, is less awkward, since she is sitting on your lap and can hold onto the arms of the wheelchair for support and balance. Intercourse is possible for a woman sitting in a wheelchair with her knees pulled up toward her chest and her partner between her legs (on his knees between the pedals or leaning over her). This is a useful technique if time is a factor and neither has the desire to get undressed and into a more relaxed position.

Side by side, either face-to-face or front to back with penetration of the vagina from the rear, offers other possibilities for you to think about (46, 47). You can position your legs comfortably. These positions are particularly good when you are wearing a catheter attached to a drainage bottle. They cut down on the problem of weight and balance and give a good feeling of intimacy. They also give both of you a lot of freedom of body movement and use of your hands and arms, either to help or enhance the situation.

A car will do if you do not have access to a bed or a place where you and your partner can be alone. A male paraplegic or quadriplegic can assume a variation of the sitting position, slouched down on the car seat with his partner straddling him. This gives a lot of support in the back and trunk muscles and gives the woman quite a bit of freedom of movement. Oral-genital stimulation can easily be done by having your partner simply lie down on the seat with his or her back and shoulders against the door. (Caution is advised on well-traveled roads.)

47

If you are a male paraplegic or quadriplegic and you and your partner like the option of penile-vaginal penetration, but you are not always capable of an erection, you might want to consider the possibility of using a penis stiffener or dildo. A stiffener is usually made of a formed piece of hard rubber that fits over the penis and holds it stiff enough for penetration. Another type of stiffener can be surgically implanted in the penis to produce a constantly erect penis, and there are others that are in the experimental stage; if you are interested, you should consult your physician about the necessary surgery. A dildo is an artificial penis, usually made of semihard rubber, which can be strapped on above the penis or held in the hand (48). It enables you to give your partner the sensation of penetration and penile-vaginal stimulation.

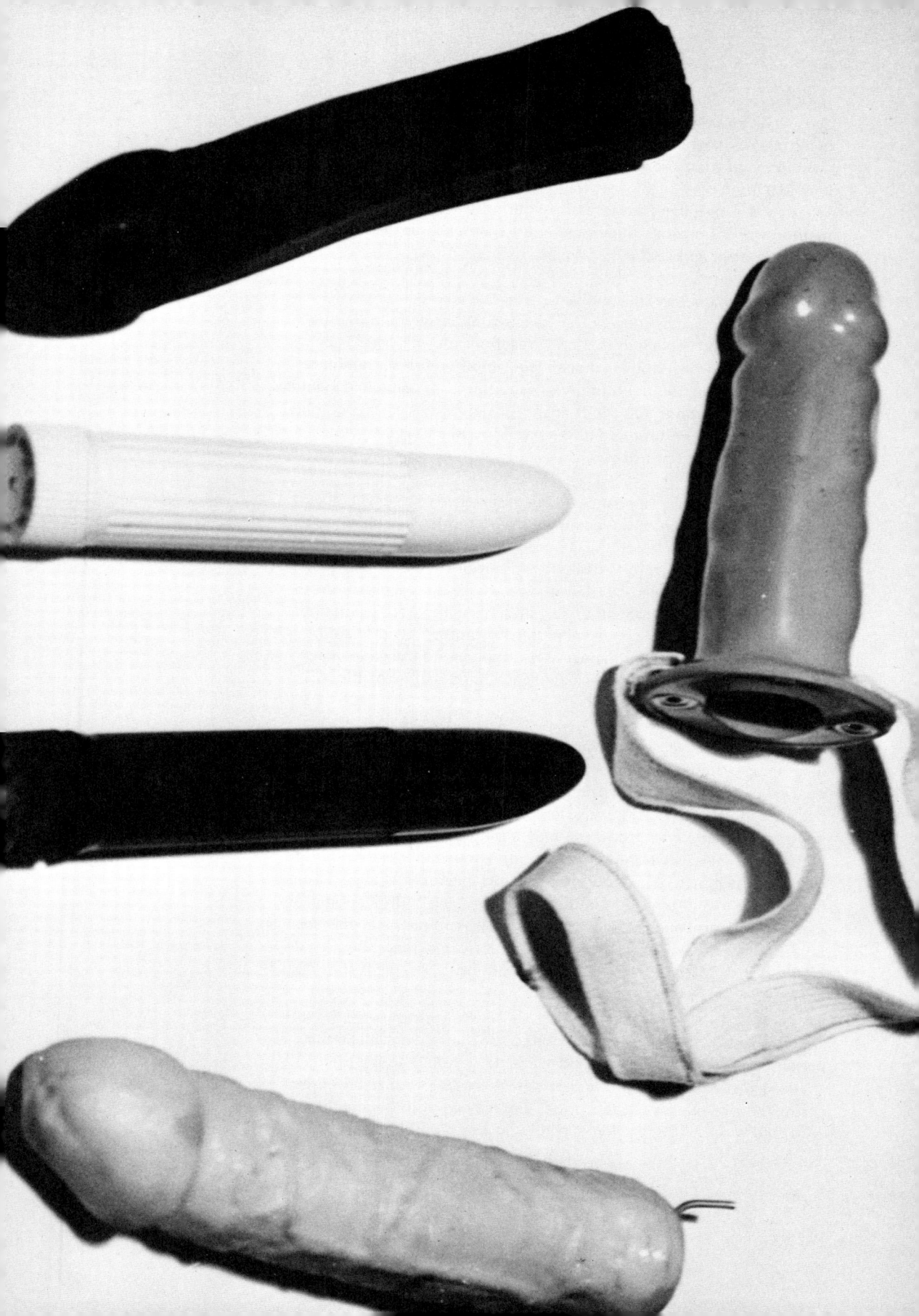

In order to get better body motion, you may want to consider a water bed. A feature of the water bed that is valued by some paraplegics and quadriplegics, particularly those with a high-level injury, is that the motion of the mattress gives them more body movement during foreplay and intercourse. Another way to achieve more movement during intercourse is by taking advantage of your muscle spasms. While this method works for some, others say that a spasm causes them to lose bladder control and causes men to lose their erection.

As we have said before, the ability to fantasize an orgasm can be developed to an intense degree. By keeping the lights on in the room, using mirrors to enable you to see the reactions of your partner better, talking about the sensations you can feel, amplifying them, and integrating all of them in your mind, you can achieve an enjoyable mental orgasm. The methods you try or adapt for your own use depend only on your physical limitations and the options you and your partner decide are best for both of you.

If leakage of a urinary appliance or the occurrence of a bowel movement during intercourse is a seemingly insurmountable problem, you and your partner can lessen the chance of an accident by using a little care in your positioning. If a leak does occur or if you happen to have a bowel movement, we know that it is demoralizing and pretty much of a turn-off. You could fake a heart attack and hope for sympathy. However, like the Boy Scouts, we prefer the motto, "Be prepared." The occasion when it does happen is not the time to introduce your partner to the possibilities of accidents and hope that he or she will understand.

There are a few special problems that you as a female paraplegic or quadriplegic should remember. When an able-bodied woman is sexually aroused by the physical things that are happening, her vagina usually becomes moist. If your injury is complete, your mental attitude cannot affect this moistness, and you may have to rely on assistance for lubrication. The penis itself does not emit enough lubricating fluid to maintain the moisture necessary for comfortable lovemaking. If you have both a loss of sensation in the genital area and a lubrication problem, you will probably have to ask your partner to notice if your vagina is getting too dry for ease and comfort. Lubricants should be kept handy if the problem does arise and the motion of the penis starts to chafe the walls of your vagina.

If you wear a catheter and desire intercourse during your menstrual period, you run the risk of a bladder infection should your catheter chafe against either you or your partner. If you do wish to have intercourse during your menstrual period, you may want to douche first with cold water. This usually stops the flow of blood for a while.

If you are a spinal cord—injured female having sex with a fertile male, and you wear a catheter while the male wears a condom for contraception, he should be careful, since it might rupture and leak from rubbing against the catheter. You should consult with your own physician as to the method or methods of birth control that would be the best for you. Pregnancy can readily occur in the paraplegic or quadriplegic woman. With a few exceptions, prenatal care and childbirth are normal. (For more details about birth control and pregnancy, see *contraception* and *pregnancy* in the Glossary.)

If you are not using a catheter, it would be a good idea to empty your bladder as well as you can before you get into position for sexual activity. You may find that the penis's penetration of the vagina, as well as the action of intercourse itself, puts pressure on your bladder and causes you to urinate. With forethought, use of your imagination, and care in your positioning, there should be nothing to keep you from assuming any position that you and your partner prefer or choose to try.

5 Oral-Genital and Manual Stimulation

If your eyes are the windows of your soul, then your mouth must be the expression of it.
— Rubaiyat of Omar Khayam

A commonly used means of sexual expression for the spinal cord–injured person is the use of the mouth to excite and give pleasure to his or her partner (49–56). You may find that you receive more pleasure with this option, partly because your lips and tongue, which have not been impaired by your injury, are more sensitive to touch and temperature than any other part of your body. In addition, the sensations you receive from the smell, taste, and texture of your partner's skin are heightened and could be quite a turn-on for you. The act of kissing and caressing many areas of your partner's body in a sensuous, tender way will enhance the feelings of togetherness. When you and your partner are caressing and using your mouths on each other at the same time, or even if one of you is passive, the sensations can be tremendously pleasing. The sensations you receive from your partner's tongue caressing or sucking a sensitive area, such as your ear, neck, wrist, breast, or genital area, can be transposed to another part of your body that has less sensitivity.

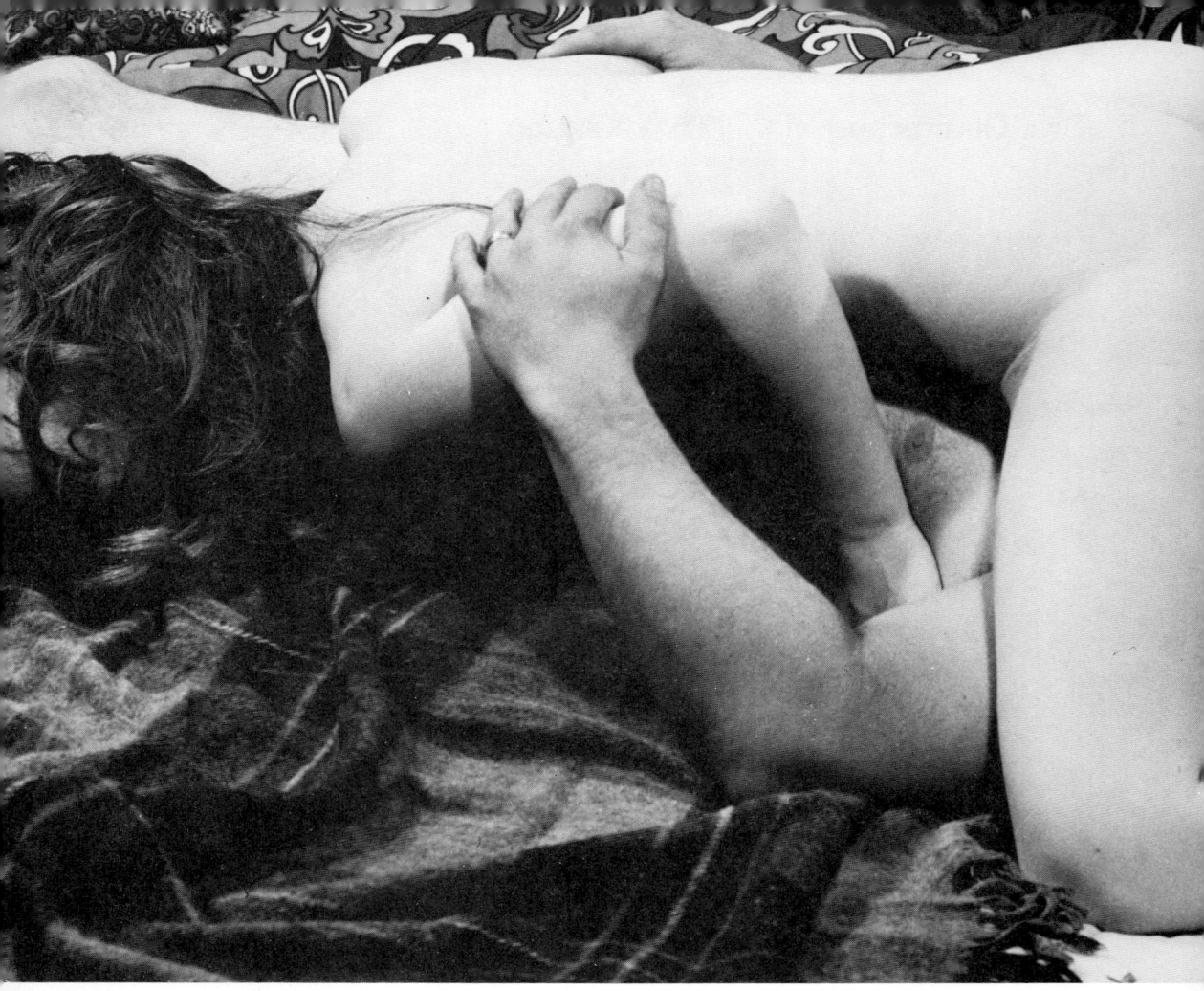
49

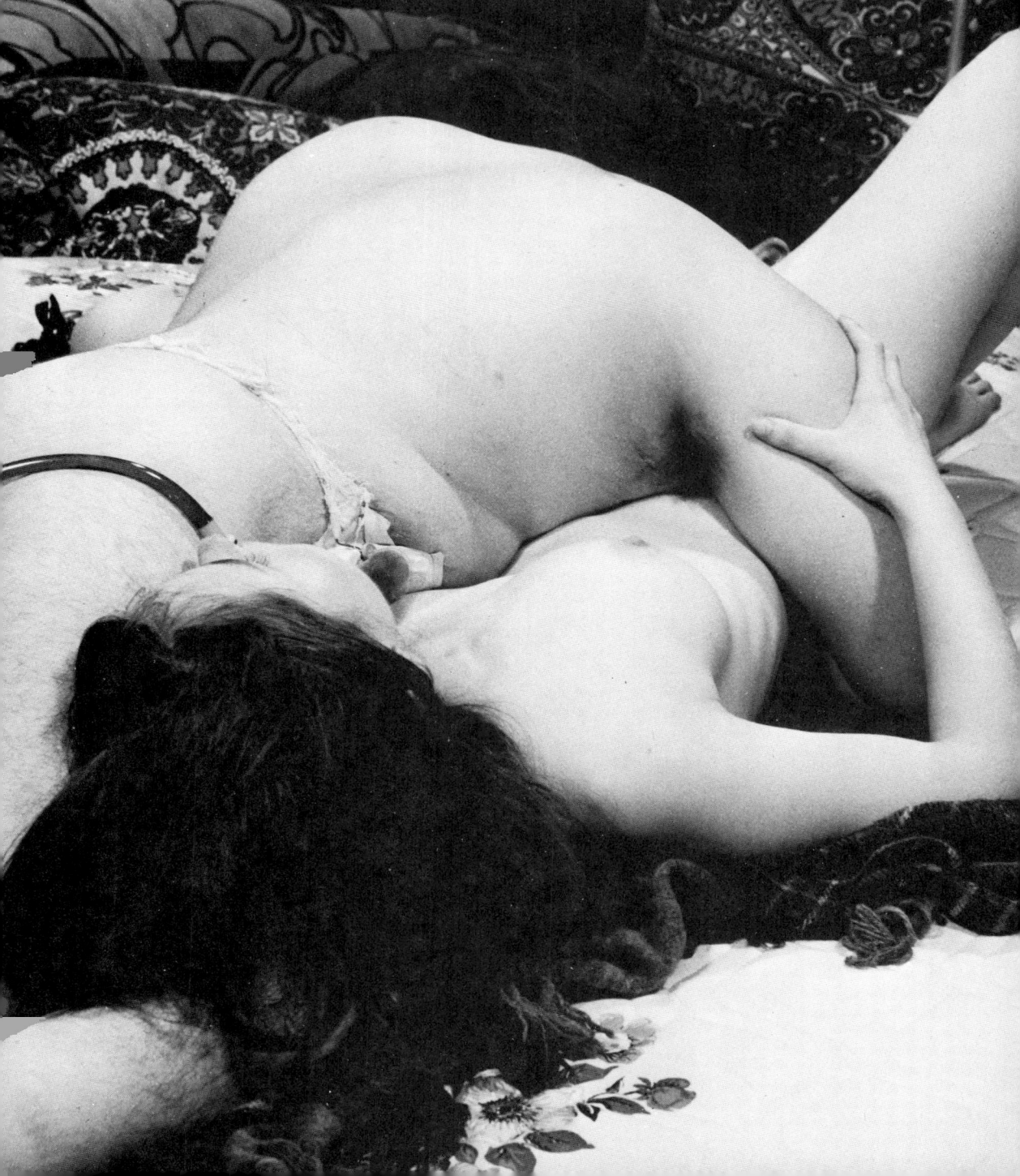

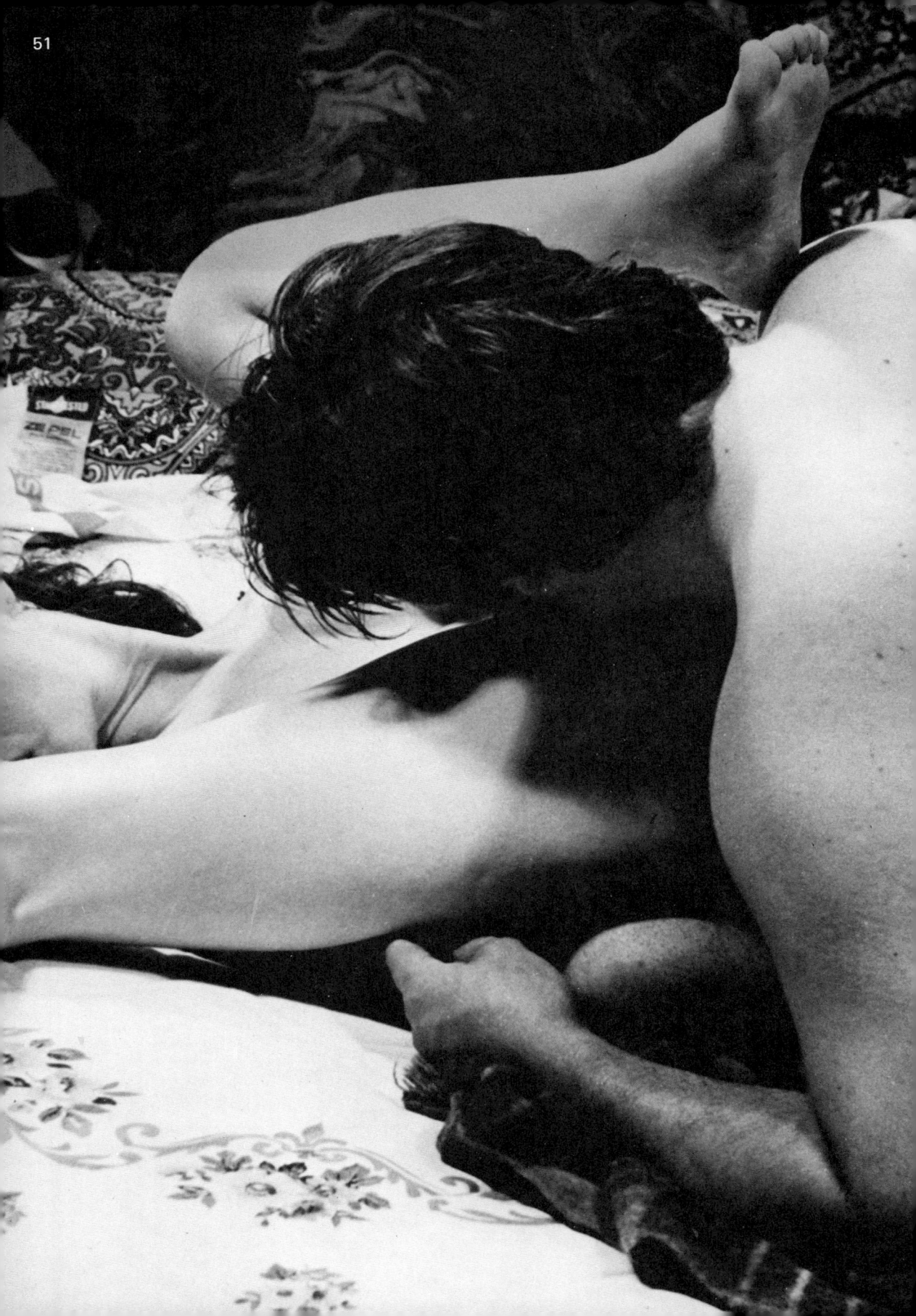

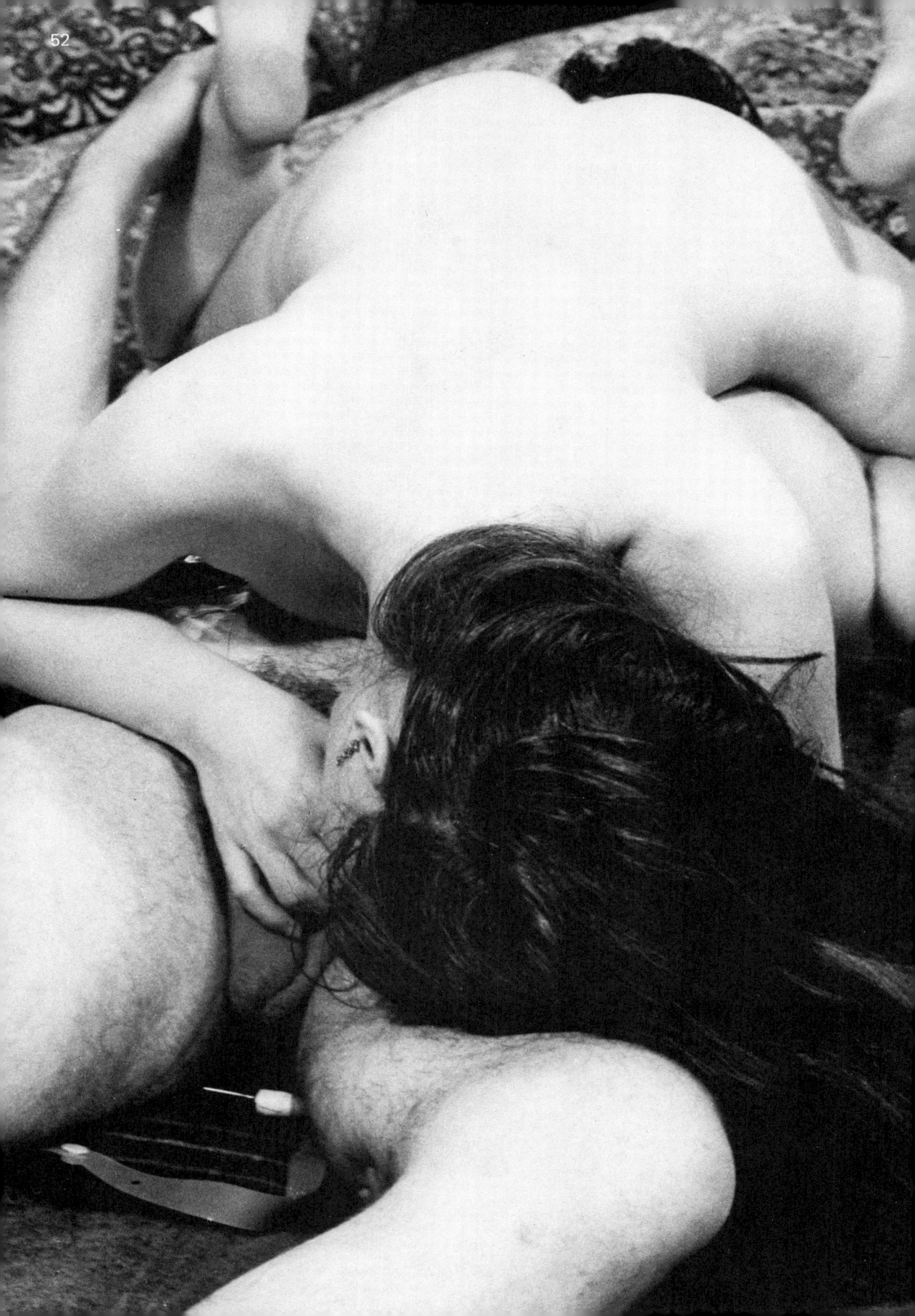

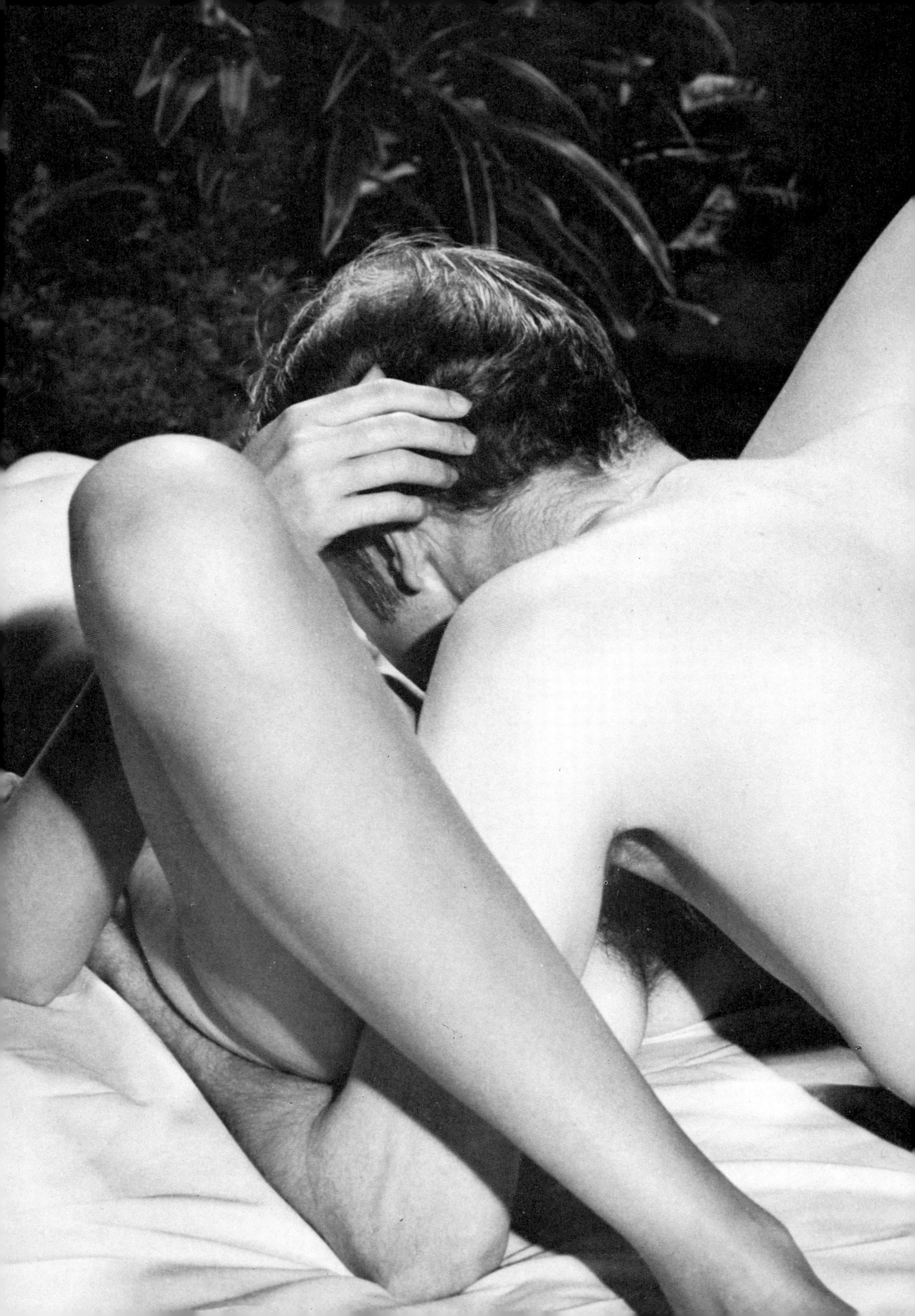

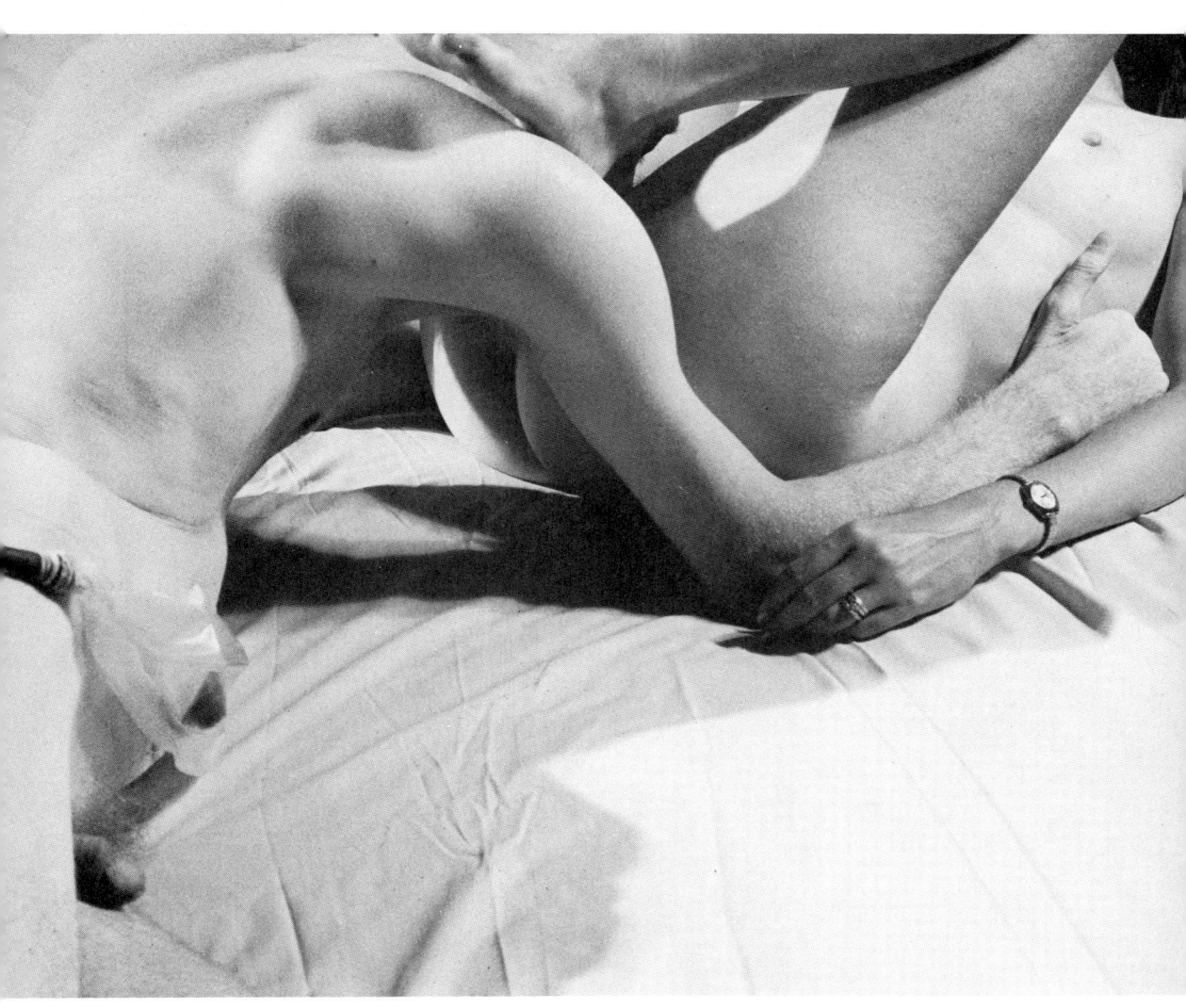

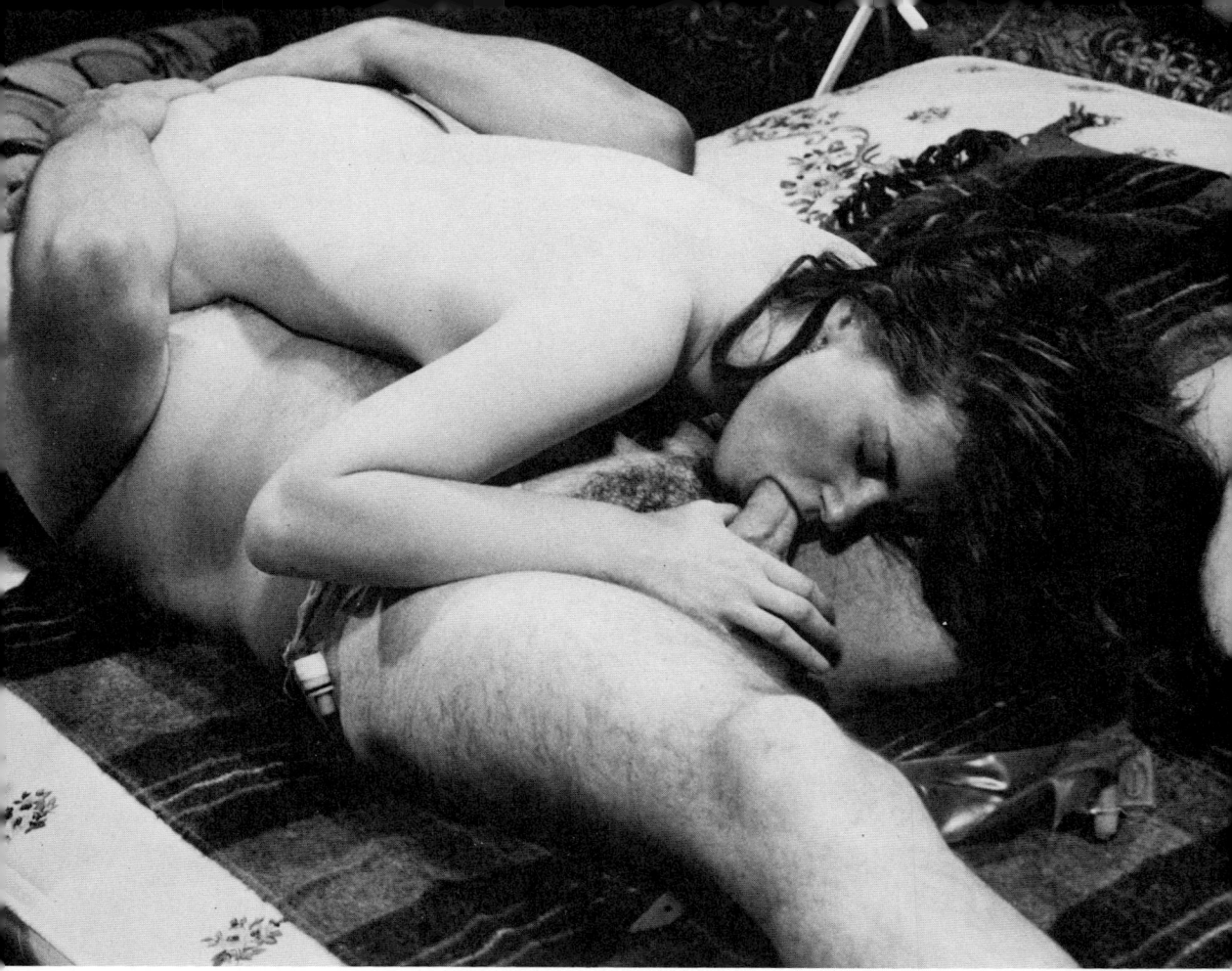

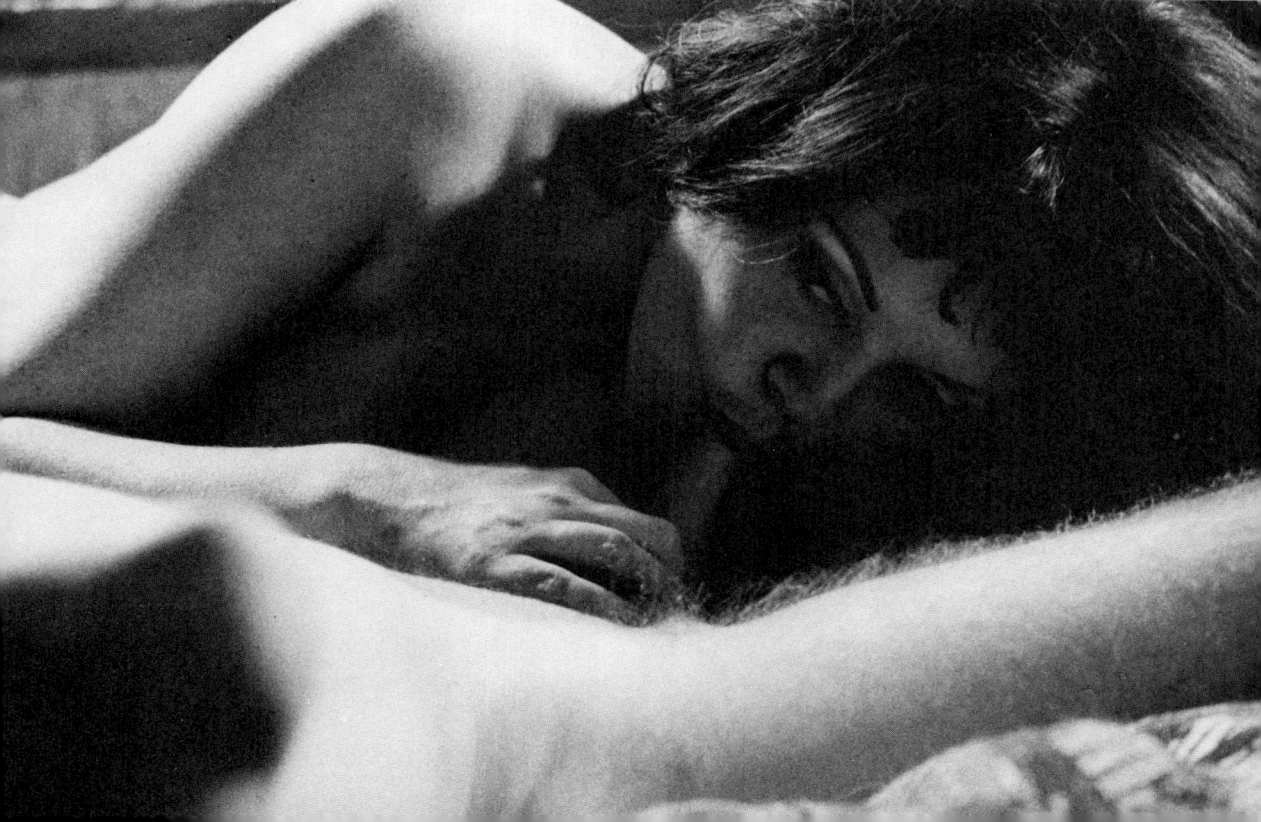

Oral-genital sexual activity can be done mutually by two partners who position themselves in a way that make each partner's genitals easily available to the other's mouth (49, 52).

Because of your difficulty in changing positions quickly, your partner might have to be the one who does the shifting and the positioning. Either through your verbal directions or the refined communication of touch, you can develop a style of lovemaking that is beautifully tender and passionate.

Whether you use oral stimulation for transposing sensation, for arousal in foreplay, or if you and your partner simply enjoy it, remember that any part of the body can be made clean enough for oral contact. So do not be hesitant to try oral stimulation in any way you may want to. It can be enjoyable and fun for you and your partner. Keep in mind that the penis and vagina are highly sensitive to receiving pleasure and that the hands with their high degree of dexterity and the mouth with its great sensitivity, have a great capacity for giving pleasure. Paraplegics and quadriplegics who choose this enjoyable option find that the old jokes and myths that surround oral-genital sex are just that and have little validity.

Each of us receives taste and smell in a different way. Everyone has his or her own individual scent and taste. As you know, the odor from any part of the body is caused by normal secretions of the skin. Once the area is clean, there is no odor other than the natural scent of the individual. In a reasonably clean and healthy person, the vagina or penis has no more harmful germs than, and is not very different in taste from, a person's mouth. It should be noted, however, that in some instances the mouth can transmit a type of yeast infection to the genital area that can cause an irritating rash. The soap, oil, or other substance you use on each other will add to or change the taste you receive when you use oral stimulation.

The degree of pleasure that couples experience in oral-genital sex differs a great deal, depending on their own preferences. To include everyone in a general statement on the satisfaction that this sexual activity offers, would be unfair. We can state, however, that in our experience most married couples have used oral-genital stimulation as part of their sexual expression. Some men do not enjoy cunnilingus (in which the male stimulates the woman, perhaps to climax, by use of his mouth and tongue on her clitoris) because they do not like the smell and taste. But the majority of males enjoy it and derive great pleasure from it. They would be likely to say that a woman's orgasm has no particular taste, except that of a warm, wet mingling of their own wet mouth taste with the body taste of their partner. Most women find the cunnilingus orgasm just as intense and satisfying as an orgasm with penile-vaginal stimulation and enjoy it as much as the male enjoys fellatio, in which the woman uses her mouth on her partner's penis. Cunnilingus is a sexual activity that can be engaged in by almost everyone if so desired. The quadriplegic man who can raise himself on his elbows can use the male dominant position, but if he is unable to do so, his partner can position herself over him while he lies on his back (53, 54).

A woman can have mixed emotions about fellatio (55, 56). She may or may not like it immediately, depending on past experiences that she has had. Women who have orally stimulated the male to ejaculation have varied opinions on the taste of sperm. The opinions range from "no particular taste" to "sweet," "very salty," or "something like diluted vinegar." However, they usually do agree that seminal fluid emitted before ejaculation tastes salty and that the consistency of the sperm varies a great deal. A woman who has not tasted it should not try, the first time, to take the entire amount that is ejaculated but should begin by tasting a small amount that could be diluted with the saliva in her mouth. Oil or any other lubricant also would work. A good principle for a man to follow is not to try to force his penis down his partner's throat and thus gag her, but to let her take as much as she desires into her mouth. Also, if he does not let her keep her head free so she can disengage when she wants, she could get that pinned-down, trapped feeling that might turn her off for the next time. Those who do try oral-genital sex usually like the responses of their partner and derive a great deal of pleasure and satisfaction from it. So, find your own methods, use your imagination, enjoy; in short, have fun. Who knows? If you try it, you might like it.

Manual stimulation of your partner is the use of any part of your body other than your genitals or mouth to stimulate and please your partner (33, 57–59). There are many parts of your body that can be used to penetrate the vagina or envelop the penis in order to stimulate your partner to orgasm. A finger, thumb, wrist, elbow, or knee can be enough of a protrusion to stimulate the clitoris. A hand, an armpit, or pressed together breasts or buttocks can envelop a penis. It is rubbing and stroking the sensitive areas of the penis and the vagina and clitoris that bring a man or woman to orgasm. Depending on your ability for movement, you can let your partner supply the rhythm and motion or increase your enjoyment by trying it yourself.

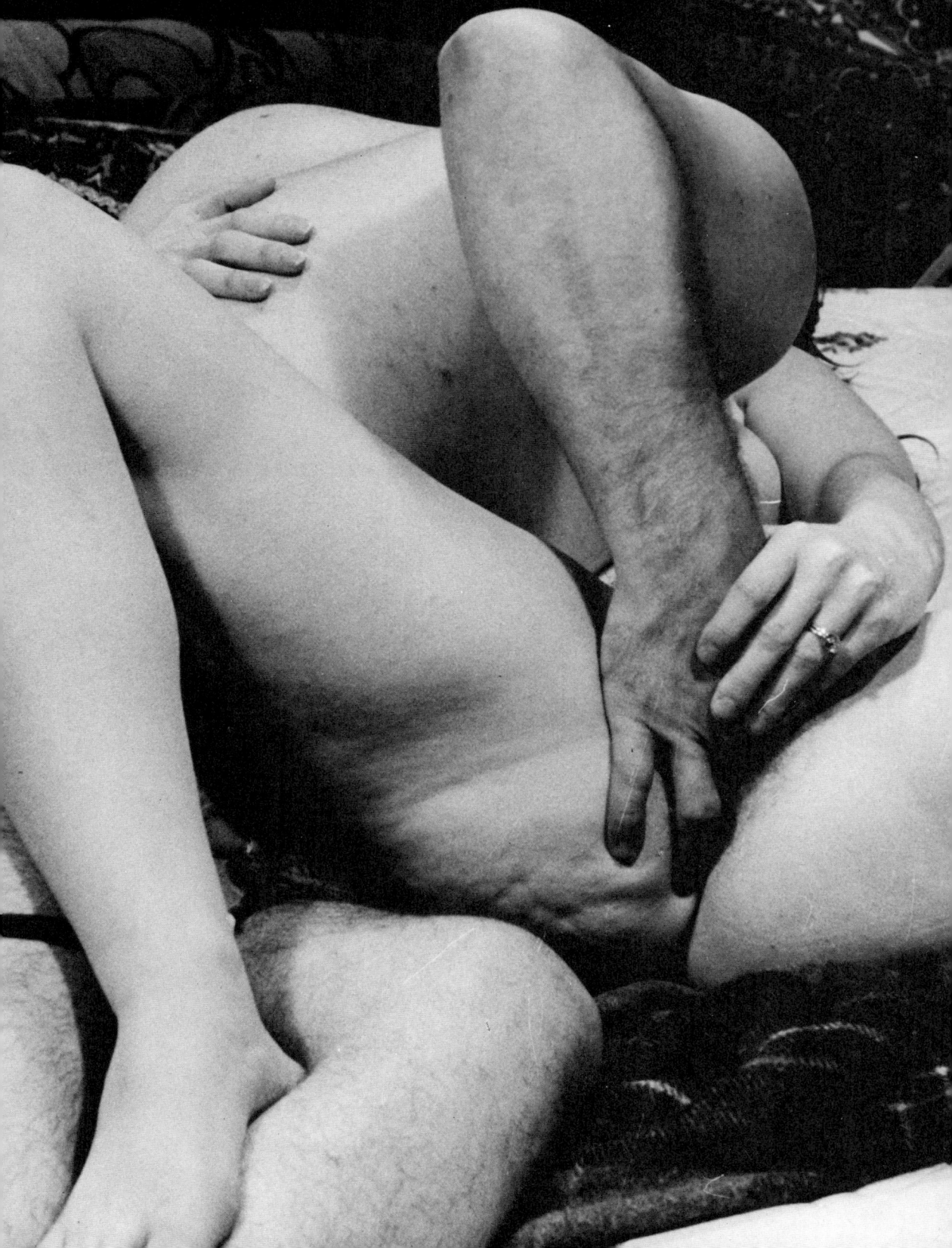

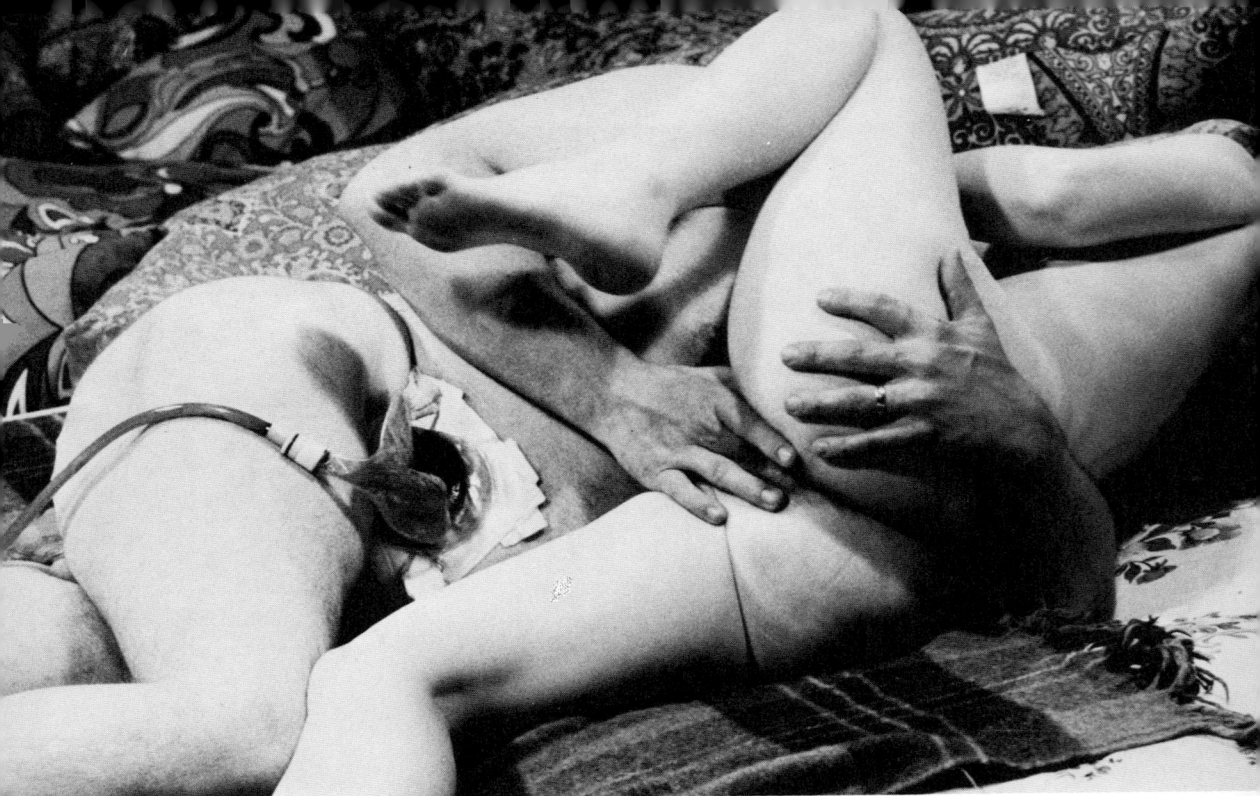

59

If your injury hinders your participation, you can use a vibrator, holding it in your hand or mouth, or another mechanical means, such as a muscle spasm to provide movement. The battery-powered electrical vibrator is an especially convenient and pleasure-giving device for stimulating a woman's genitals. The device shown in photographs 60 through 62 is lightweight and can be managed even with hands that are weakened by quadriparesis. Only your imagination limits the methods you can try. Using visual aids such as light or mirrors to see your partner's reaction, empathizing with his or her sensations, using mental techniques that you have developed, or fantasizing can please and satisfy your partner as well as yourself.

Remember, satisfying your partner should add to your satisfaction; it should not become your only goal to the exclusion of your own satisfaction.

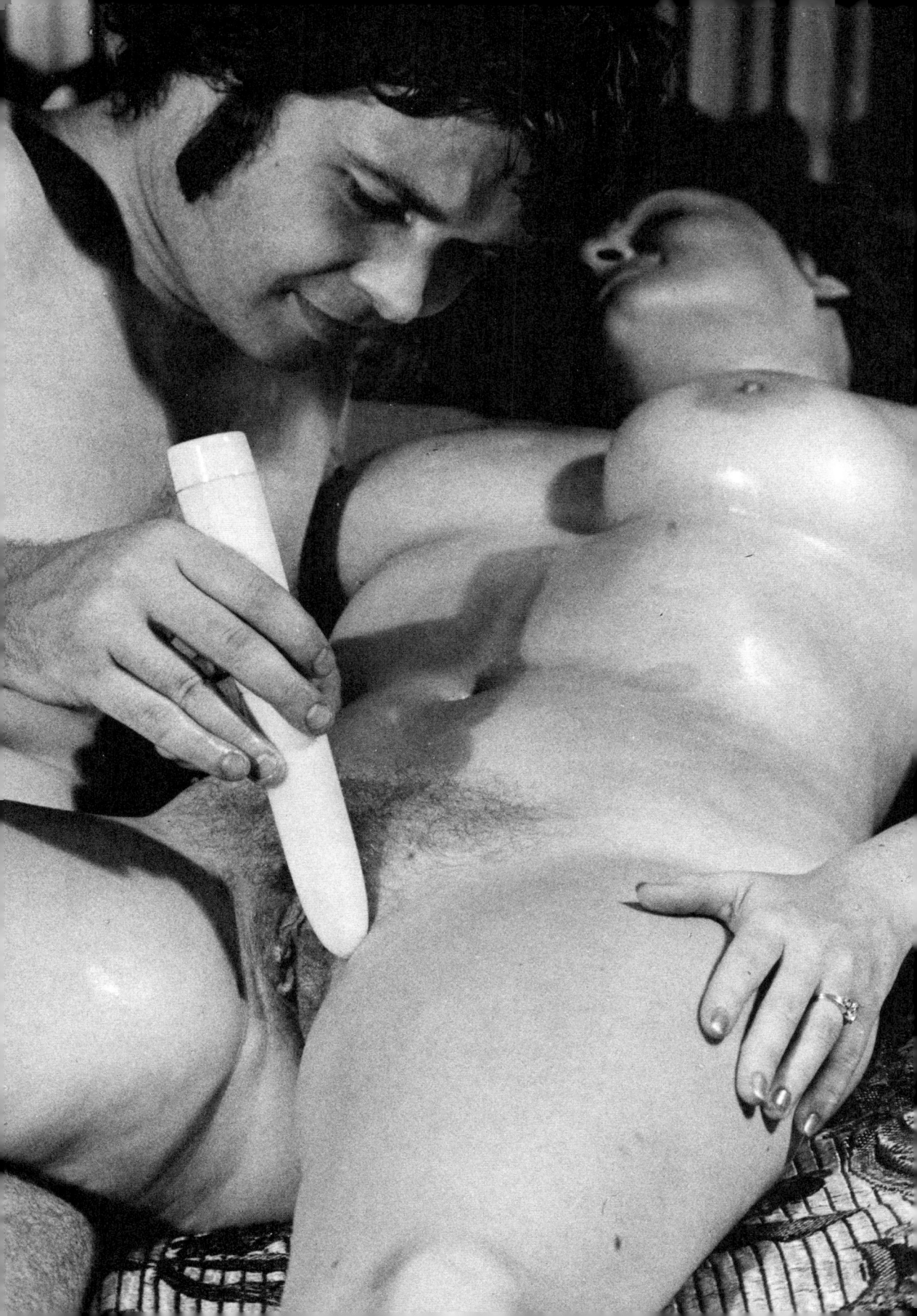

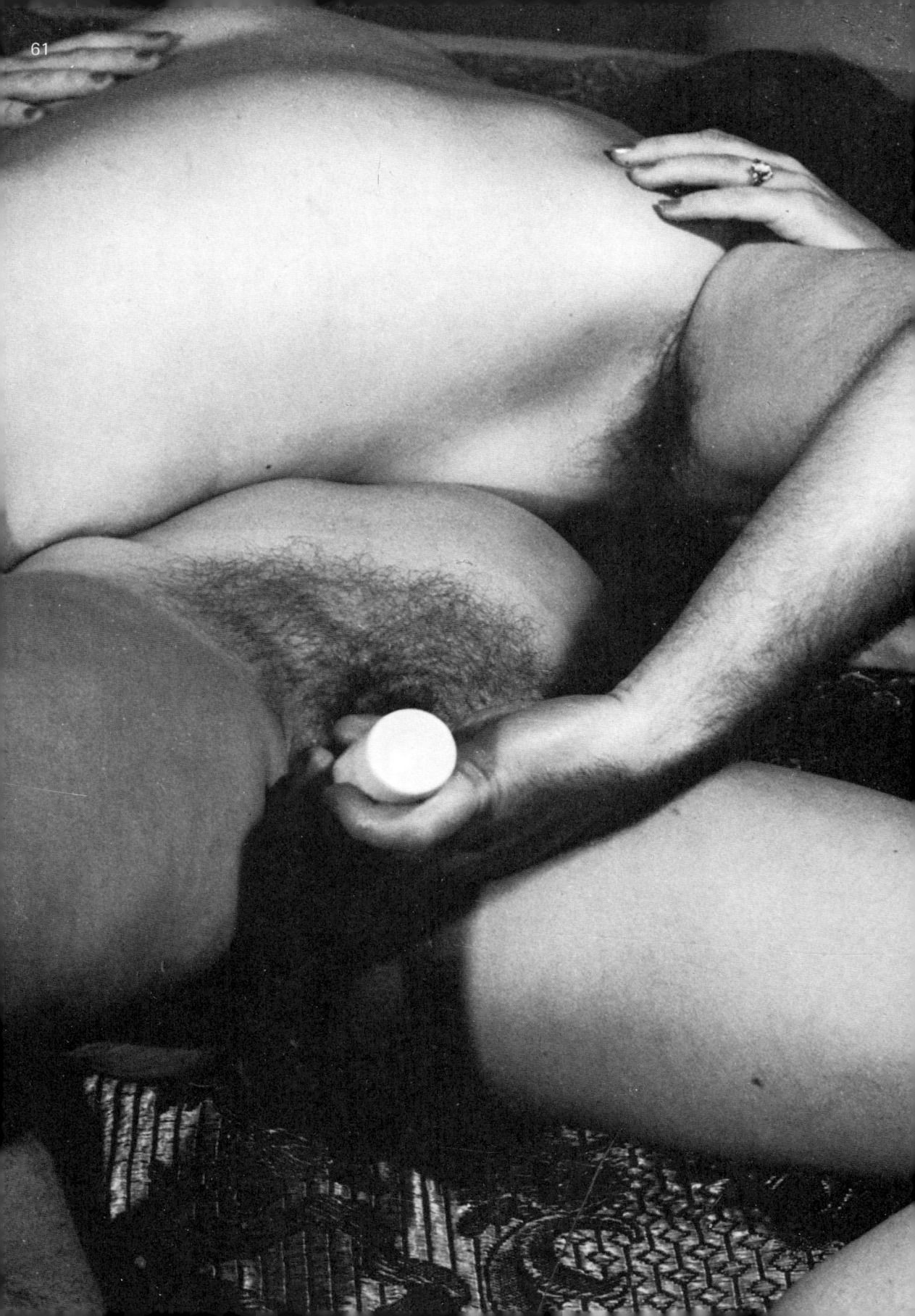

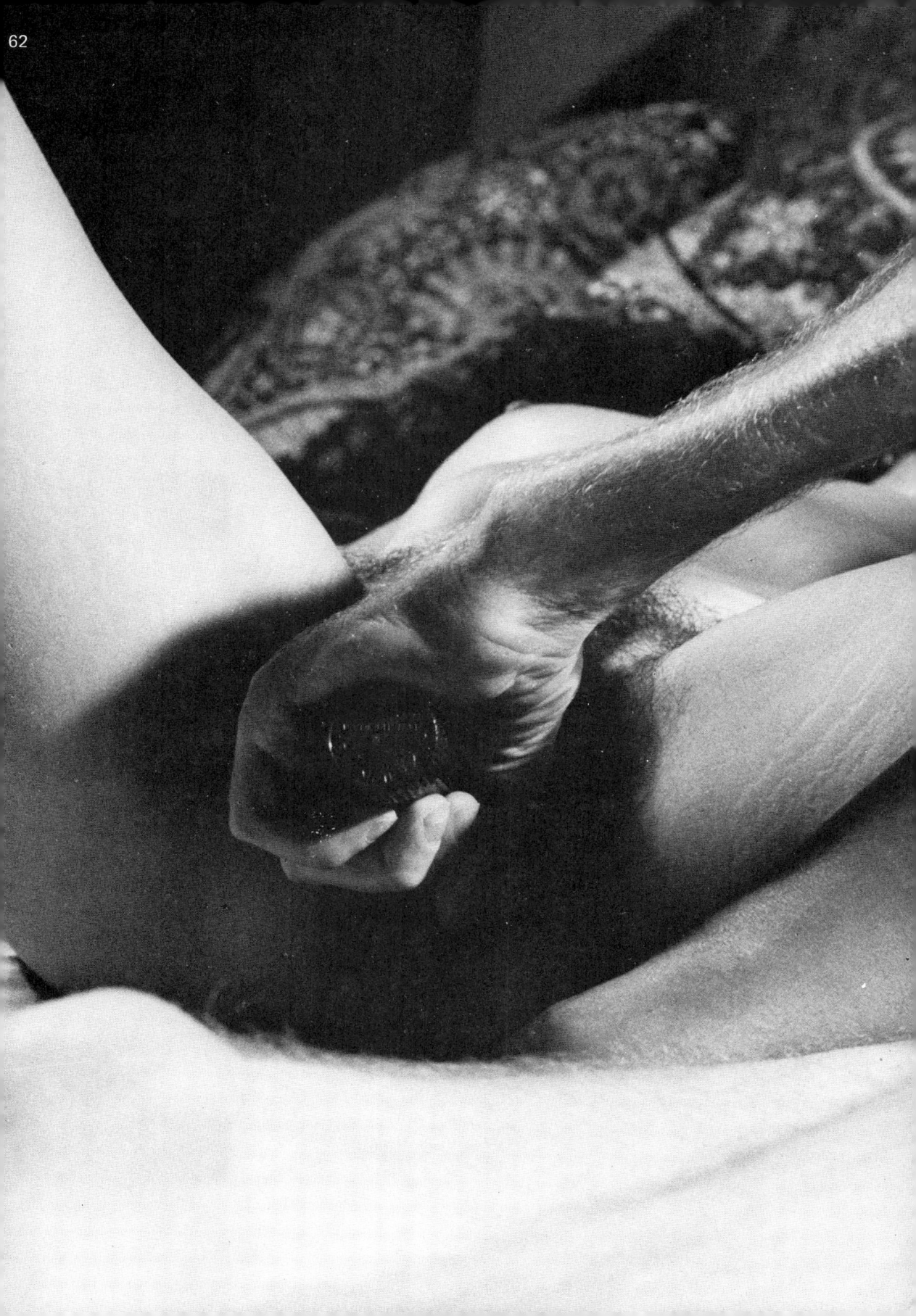

Every couple enjoys a different experience when relaxing, or "coming down," after high sexual arousal. You may find that the pleasure of lying together after lovemaking can be a warm and touching experience (63). Whether you hug or gently squeeze each other, talk about feelings, or just remember the mutual sensations, you may find that taking the time to hold and stroke your partner will greatly enhance your sexual intimacy (64).

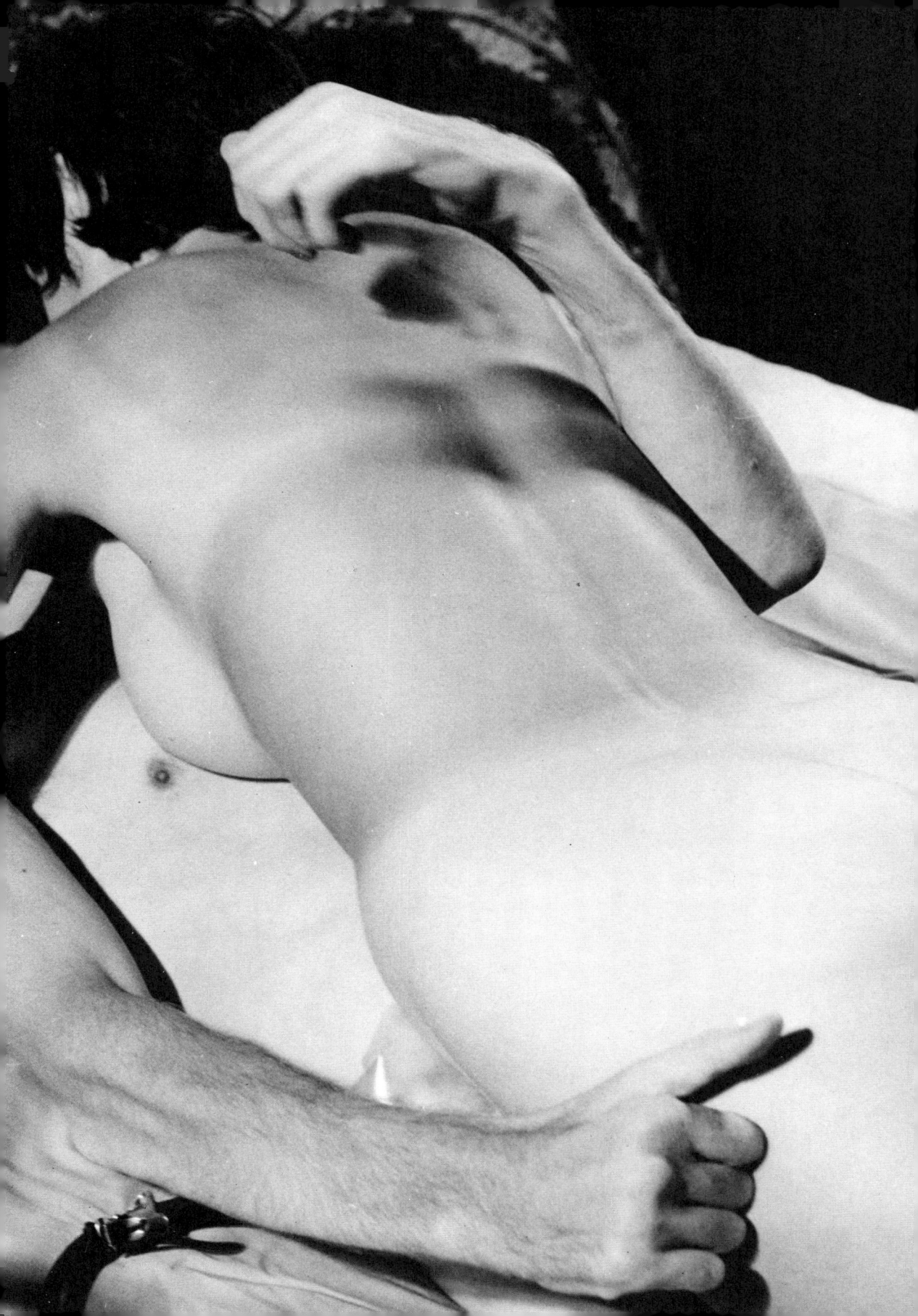

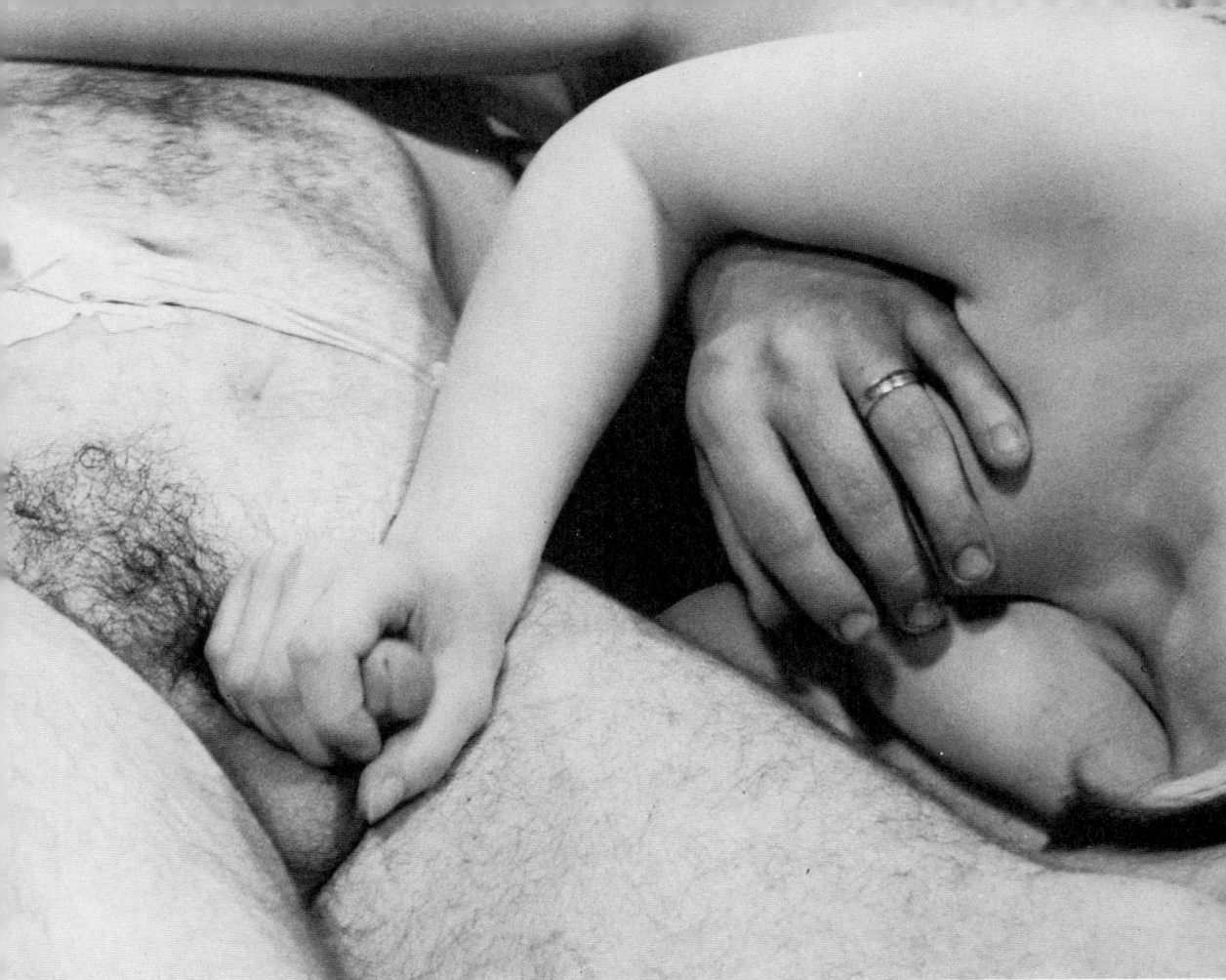
64

During the course of your relationship you may have doubts that threaten your confidence or general well-being, and you may ask yourself, "Am I good enough?" or "Is my partner really happy and satisfied?" Questions such as these and other doubts that you may have can only be answered by you and your partner.

Unspoken doubts can undermine your confidence and affect your ability to be a satisfying and inventive partner. You may try so hard that your partner will be turned off with your "performance trip," which will even further affect your self-confidence. Finding out how your partner feels and what is pleasing to both of you through open and honest communication (65) can go a long way toward answering some of the questions and self-doubts you may have. Talking in such a manner can increase your confidence in yourself and help strengthen the relationship between you and your partner.

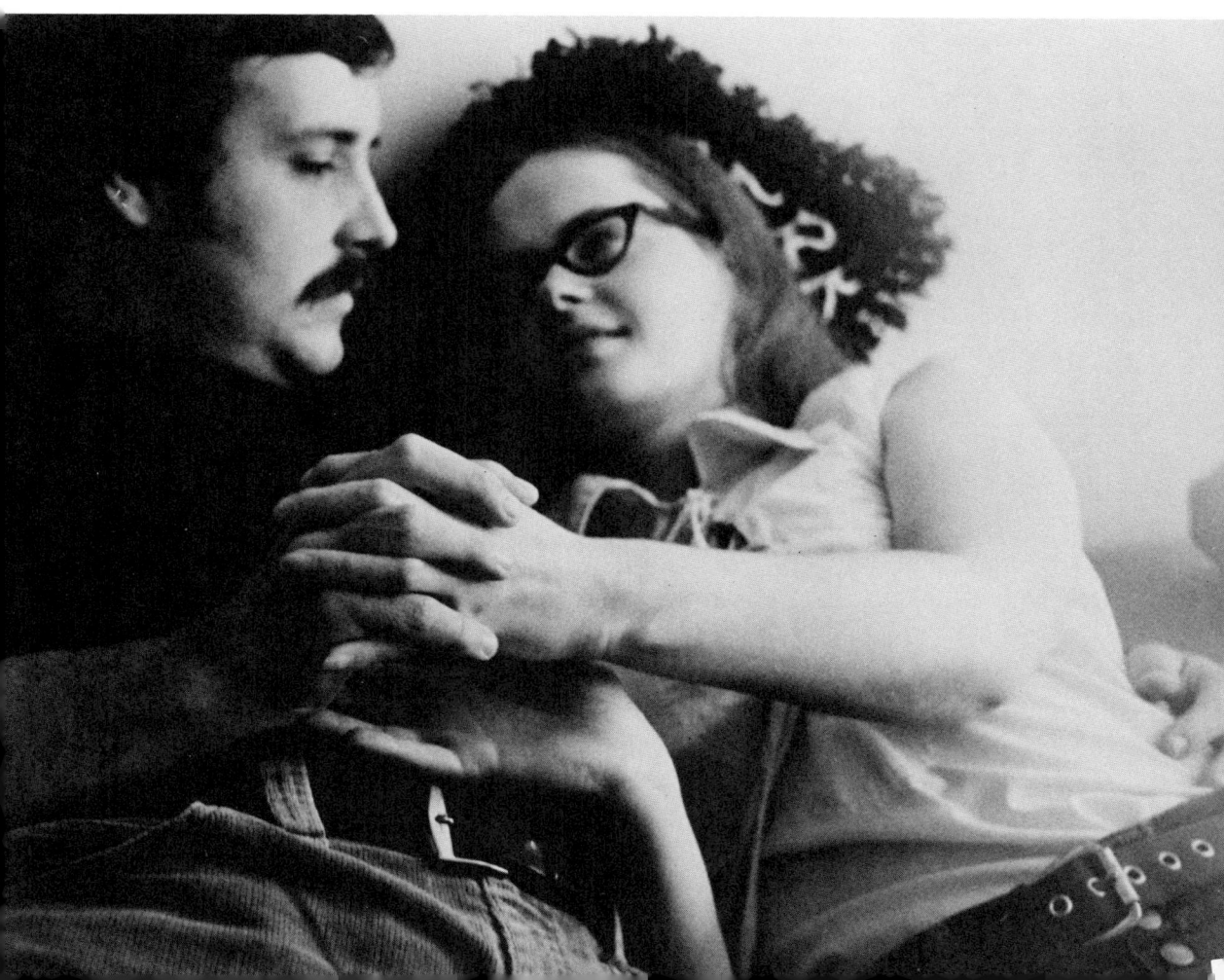

Try to remember two things: (1) Be yourself and let things happen at whatever pace is good for both of you. (2) Enjoy yourself.

While it is true that your sexual expression is usually shared with another person, the responsibility and the decision to be and remain a sexual being is and must be yours alone. Perhaps you may not choose to participate in acts of sex. Sex is, after all, just a part of your total sexuality, and choosing not to engage in sex acts does not mean that you are not sexual. Whatever choice you make, try to think of your ability, not your disability. Feel good about your choice and about yourself. Show people who you are, not what you appear to be.

Glossary

ABD pad A disposable, clean gauze pad that can be kept close by for wiping or cleaning up.

alternate sensation A feeling or sensation from a part of the body that has sensation and that can be substituted for a sensation that has been lost in another part of the body.

sensory amplification Thinking about and concentrating on a physical sensation until the sensation becomes more and more intense.

appliances

    muscle support appliances These include back braces, splints, leg braces, and mechanical devices that are used to support or assist the normal function of a muscle.

    urine-collection appliances (rig, gizmo, bag) Most paraplegics and quadriplegics suffer loss of bladder control and must use a device or tubing to collect and store body wastes. Some types of catheters in use are:

        ileostomy or **diversion** A surgical opening on the side or front of the abdomen connecting with a bag that collects the urine.

indwelling or **Foley catheter** A tube inserted into the bladder through the urethra.

condom or **Texas catheter** A latex, plastic, or rubber sheath that fits around and is secured by tape or elastic to the outside of the penis.

Whatever type of catheter is used, it is connected to a rubber or plastic bag by a short tube so that the urine can be contained and be emptied periodically. When a catheter is used at night or when a person is in bed, a longer piece of tubing connected to a large bottle or other container can sometimes be more convenient because of the smaller capacity of a collection bag.

autonomic hyperreflexia A condition caused by high spinal cord injury, resulting in a rise in blood pressure, sweating, flushing, and a painful headache in those with injury above the fourth thoracic vertebra (T-4). (For additional details, see *pregnancy*.)

bowel training As part of the rehabilitation process, spinal cord—injured people are trained to regulate their bowel movements to a certain part of the day or to stimulate a conditioned response of the rectum by touching around the rectal opening or using other types of stimulation.

contraception If you are a man with a spinal cord injury and you are unable to have an orgasm, or ejaculate, then it is not necessary for you to take measures for pregnancy prevention. You are infertile, as we have indicated previously, and you need not be concerned about causing an unwanted pregnancy. If you are a woman with a spinal cord injury, however, contraception remains as important for you now as it was before your spinal cord injury. The chances are excellent that you are just as fertile as you were before the injury. Thus, if you want to avoid pregnancy, you will have to be just as careful as ever. Your choice of contraceptive techniques, however, is influenced by your spinal cord injury. Prior to your injury you may have had your choice of the pill, intrauterine coils, the diaphragm, foams, or condoms worn by your partner. Now that you are a paraplegic or quadriplegic woman, you must think twice about these methods. As you probably know, the pill is known to increase the chance of blood clots in the veins of the legs and pelvis; the effects of the pill together with those of spinal cord injury, can increase the chance of thrombophlebitis (inflammation and clots) in a blood vessel. Since thrombophlebitis can be medically dangerous to you if a clot from the vessel travels to your lung (a pulmonary embolus), you must seek the advice of your doctor before using the pill for contraception.

The coil, or the intrauterine device, which is inserted into a woman's uterus to prevent pregnancy, is very effective for most women but carries somewhat of a risk for paralyzed women. If you have lost sensation in your pelvis, you may not be able to feel the coil should it begin to become loose or penetrate the wall of the uterus, as it sometimes does during complications. Again, you should seek the advice of your doctor, who should be familiar with the use of these devices as well as with spinal cord injuries.

Quadriplegic women may have difficulty in manipulating the diaphragm for insertion in the vagina. The use of foam or jelly may be difficult for some women if spinal cord injury has limited the use of their hands. In many of these instances, however, the woman can receive help from her partner if he is able-bodied or has good use of his hands.

We would like to conclude with a few words about parenthood. Some spinal cord—injured people may have been advised to avoid pregnancy because of their injury. It has been our experience, however, that adults who wish to raise children should be encouraged to consider doing so. However, as in the case of all considerations about your life-style after spinal cord injury, you should give careful thought to the influence of paralysis on your ability to perform whatever task it is you undertake, whether it be raising children or something else. For spinal cord—injured as well as for able-bodied people the ability to have or raise children may be very important and should not be dismissed lightly. For many spinal cord—injured men who cannot ejaculate and therefore cannot fertilize their partners, adoption may be an answer. If you have questions about this, you should seek advice from your doctor about your ability to fertilize, conceive, or raise children, or about adoption. We have heard of women who have been cautioned against raising children by well-meaning doctors who simply do not understand spinal cord injury. We know of women who have had children and raised them, either adopted or natural-born, and done a superb job, despite their spinal cord injury. The experienced paraplegic or quadriplegic adult understands his or her own physical limitations and should be able to work out what necessary assistance and support might be needed to manage a family. Obviously, the involvement of your partner in these discussions is essential.

Credé's method A technique to empty the bladder by applying pressure directly to the bladder area with the hands.

cunnilingus The act of stimulating a woman's vulva, clitoris, or vagina with the mouth or tongue.

dildo An artificial penis, usually made of plastic or rubber, which can be solid or can be hollow, allowing the male to place it over his penis with the aid of a strap or harness.

dominant position (male or female) The position used by two partners engaging in sexual intercourse in which either the male or the female is on top.

fellatio The act of stimulating a man's penis or scrotum with the mouth or tongue.

fertility One method of obtaining sperm in the spinal cord—injured male involves the injection of certain chemical compounds into the area of the spinal cord. These chemicals affect nerves in the spinal cord, produce contractions of the muscular tissues of the man's genital organs, and thereby cause him to expel sperm. Often, however, due to spasticity of muscles in the pelvis, the sperm are forced upward and backward into the bladder rather than up and outward through the penis. Where there is success in forcing sperm out of the penis, the sperm is then collected by a doctor and placed in the woman's vagina, where it may cause her to become pregnant.

Electrical stimulation of the man's internal sex organs has also been successfully tried in a few cases. In this method, an electrical probe about the size of a finger or thumb is inserted several inches into the man's rectal opening. In this position it touches parts of the man's sexual organs that contain sperm and causes the organs to squeeze and contract. This squeezing causes the sperm contained in them to be squirted along the tubes between the internal organs and either the penis or the bladder. In some cases the spasticity in the pelvis muscles forces the sperm up and backward into the bladder. In other cases sperm may be squirted up, forward, and out through the penis. Unfortunately for most spinal cord—injured men, the sperm collected by this method are not entirely normal. The sperm are fewer in number (normally, thousands of sperm are in each drop of a man's ejaculate) and are usually not normal in their shape or in their ability to wiggle and move about. Because of these differences, the sperm may not be able to fertilize an egg.

Kegel exercises These exercises are designed to strengthen the pubococcygeus muscle and surrounding musculature. This muscle and its adjuncts help to control the urinary outlet; however, they also appear to be associated with the capacity for receiving sensory pleasure in the vaginal and clitoral areas. Women who have practiced Kegel exercises for a period of time report increased muscle tonus in the vagina, ability to constrict the vagina voluntarily, and increased capacity for achieving orgasm.

In order for the woman to learn which muscles are involved and how to contract them, she should first stand facing the toilet as though she were a man about to urinate. Then she should pretend to release a stream of urine and abruptly inhibit it before the first drops are released. The contraction involved in inhibiting the stream is the basic maneuver of Kegel exercises. Once having experienced the method of contracting, the woman can perform the contractions while driving an automobile, sitting, lying, or doing anything else that does not involve a great deal of moving about. She should contract the muscles, hold the contractions for a 1-2-3 (subvocal) count, release, and repeat the process. She may do as many a day as she likes — about 90 is fine. In a few weeks she will be able to constrict her vagina voluntarily with considerable strength.

Another set of exercises involves bearing down as one does during labor or during defecation. Again, a 1-2-3 count, release, and repetition is the procedure. Do a set of Kegels and a set of these exercises. They can be continued indefinitely. You might try inserting a finger in the vagina in order to feel the contractions.

manual stimulation The use of a finger, hand, or any part of the body (other than the mouth or genitals) on the genitals or another part of the body of a sexual partner.

mental orgasm Remembering or imagining (fantasizing) the sensations of physical orgasm.

oils and lubricants Each oil and lotion has its own characteristic and should be selected or tried for a special effect. One should experiment to find out what is pleasing. Each couple will develop their own preference for the type of oil or lotion that they like to use.

Most oils and lotions can be purchased at drug or department stores or in specialized bath or body shops. Oils may be mixed with a favorite scent or flavor. However, it should be noted that there are two types of oil, mineral and organic (vegetable), and that they do not mix together well.

paraplegic A person with a spinal cord injury that produces loss of feeling and voluntary muscular function of the trunk and legs.

pregnancy Pregnant women in general are more susceptible to infections in the urine, bladder and kidneys than are women who are not pregnant. This susceptibility is even greater if you are a woman with a spinal cord injury. Since the paralysis affects your bladder, sometimes requiring you to use a catheter, and since the bladder paralysis and the catheter increase your chances of getting an infection in the urine, bladder and kidneys, this susceptibility is increased even more when you become pregnant. However, doctors have antibiotics and other medication that fight these infections and help you through your pregnancy with a minimum of difficulty.

A pregnant woman with a spinal cord injury may also have difficulty in later stages of pregnancy. As you know, maintaining balance while sitting or standing is difficult for paralyzed people. This difficulty will be increased when the woman becomes pregnant and carries a moderately heavy baby in her uterus. If your spinal cord injury makes your sitting balance or transfer balance difficult, pregnancy may increase the problem. Also, able-bodied women experience some shortness of breath during the later stages of pregnancy, simply because the enlarging uterus presses against the internal organs, which in turn press upward on the breathing muscle (diaphragm) and interfere with breathing. If you are a paraplegic or a quadriplegic woman with a high-level injury, this difficulty may be somewhat increased.

Able-bodied women often experience difficulty with constipation during the later stages of pregnancy. If constipation is a problem for you, it could become worse as a result of pregnancy. The most important thing to remember is that you should put yourself in the hands of a doctor who has had experience with both pregnancy and delivery and with spinal cord injury.

Some additional problems bear mentioning. If you can feel no pain in the area of your pelvis and abdomen, then you may be unable to recognize the onset of labor pains. Some women should therefore be admitted to the hospital and watched closely by their obstetrician during the last few weeks of pregnancy in order to avoid this problem. During the final stages of labor, when the woman is being asked to bear down and strain to help the doctor deliver the baby, paraplegic and quadriplegic women are at a disadvantage. They cannot tighten their muscles in an effort to help force the baby out, and therefore the doctor has to work alone. Again, it is important for the woman to be sure she is in the hands of an obstetrician who is entirely familiar with spinal cord injury.

Perhaps the most serious problem that your spinal cord injury may cause for you during pregnancy is a condition mentioned earlier in this book, namely, autonomic hyperreflexia. Since a uterus that is contracting to push a baby out causes a great deal of stimulation to the spinal cord, delivery is one of the major causes of autonomic hyperreflexia and severe elevation of blood pressure. Many quadriplegics have experienced autonomic hyperreflexia at some time following their spinal cord injury. They recognize the severe pounding headache and the flushing that occur in association with it. Autonomic hyperreflexia is a potentially dangerous condition and needs to be dealt with immediately. High elevations of blood pressure are not good for anybody, even for short periods of time. Again, we would like to stress the fact that placing yourself in the hands of a doctor who is entirely familiar with these aspects of spinal cord injury will enable you to go through your delivery with no difficulty. The doctor can provide medication that will help control your blood pressure during delivery, and, as a result, your discomfort should be minimal.

We would like to mention some of the advantages you may experience in pregnancy and delivery as a result of your spinal cord injury. Since you probably are unable to feel pain below the level of your injury, there is no need for you to have anesthesia during delivery. Should you require a cesarean section, you may not need anesthesia for this procedure either. You may be interested to know, however, that cesarean section deliveries are no more common in women with spinal cord injury than they are in able-bodied women. If your doctor recommends cesarean section, he probably would have done so if you had been able-bodied.

quadriplegic A person with a spinal cord injury that produces loss of feeling and voluntary muscular function of the arms or hands, as well as of the trunk and legs.

reflex erection An erection of the penis that is caused by internal or external stimulation around the penis or genital area. There are some medical and surgical procedures that your doctor may recommend to control your spasticity. You should be aware that some of these procedures can cause you to lose your ability to have erections. Be sure to ask your doctor about this if you are contemplating treatment for spasticity.

stuffing technique A method by which the woman can experience the sensation of the penis in her vagina even though the male does not have an erection. It is done by using the fingers to stuff or tuck the flaccid, soft penis into the vagina. By thrusting her hips and using the muscles of her vagina, the woman can draw the soft penis into her vagina with a sort of pulling or sucking movement.

vibrators There are many types of vibrators, which offer a variety of sensations and can add a new dimension of enjoyment and pleasure. Some large department stores sell the type that fits on the hand and can be used for body or facial massage. Others, with special attachments, can be purchased without too much difficulty. Vibrators or dildos that you may wish to try may be available at your local adult book store. Catalogs can be obtained by writing to these sources:

Multi Media Resource Center
540 Powell Street
San Francisco, California 94108

Parisian Press, Inc.
30 Sheridan Street
San Francisco, California 94103

Companion Products
415 Lexington Avenue
New York, New York 10017

Index

ABD pad, 99
Aide, assistance of, 28, 31
Alternate sensation, 5, 99
Appearance, 2
  personal hygiene and, 2
Appliances, 2. *See also* Urinary drainage appliances
  attaching of, assistance by partner in, 30
  leakage of, during intercourse, 70
  for muscle support, 99
  removal of, 27, 28
Arousal, sexual, 6
  relaxing from, 6
  styles of, 35–51
Attitude toward oneself, importance of, 3
Autonomic hyperreflexia, 6, 100

Balance, maintenance of, 27
Bed. *See* Water bed
Birth control. *See* Contraception
Bladder, 2
  emptying of, before intercourse, 21, 71. *See also* Credé's method
Bowel movement, during intercourse, 2, 70
Bowel training, 100
Breasts, stimulation of, 38, 40

Car, use of, for sexual intercourse, 66
Caressing, 35, 73
Catheter
  attachment to drainage bottle, handling of, 24
  insertion of, 28
  positioning of, 14
    for intercourse, 66
      for female, 14
      for male, 13
  removal of, 28
  types of, 100
Cleanliness. *See* Hygiene
Clitoris, manual stimulation of, 84
Communication
  to eliminate self-doubt, 96
  importance of, 2, 6
  of problems, 2–3
Condom, rupture of, from catheter, 71
Condom catheter. *See* Texas catheter
Contraception, methods of, 71, 100
Credé's method, application of, 21, 101
Cunnilingus
  defined, 101
  enjoyment of, 83

Dildo, 68, 102
Diversion appliances, 14, 99
Douche, for stoppage of menstrual flow, 70

Ejaculation, 4
Erection, penile
  inability in, alternatives to
    dildo, 68
    penis stiffener, 68
    stuffing technique, 53
  reflex, 4
    defined, 105
    loss of, 51
    methods for achievement of, 46
Experimentation, importance of, 6, 48

Fantasies, 35
Fellatio, 83
  defined, 102
Female
  lubrication of, during intercourse, 70
  reproduction and, 4. *See also* Menstruation
  sexuality of, 3
Fertility, 4, 102
Foley catheter
  defined, 100
  removal and insertion of, 28
Foreplay. *See* Arousal, sexual

Goals, redefining of, 3

Hugging, 35
Hygiene
  importance of, 2, 7
  oral-genital relations and, 82

Ileostomy appliances, 99
Indwelling catheter. *See* Foley catheter
Infections, yeast, 82
Intercourse, sexual
  catheter positioning for, 13–14
  positions for, 60–66, 71
  preparation for, 71
  problems during
    bowel movement, 70
    female lubrication, 70
    rupture of condom, 71
    urinary leakage, 70
  use of car for, 66
  use of water bed for, 70
  use of wheelchair for, 66

Kegel exercises, 53, 102
Kissing, 35, 73

Lubricant(s)
  for intercourse, 70
    with catheters, 14
  types of, 43, 103
Lubrication
  of female, during intercourse, problems in, 70

Male, reproduction and, 4
Manual stimulation, 6, 40, 84, 103
Massage, 38

Masturbation, importance of, 49
Menstruation
  intercourse during, 70
  temporary cessation of, 4
Mirrors, use of, for arousal, 44
Muscle spasms, for movement during intercourse, 70

Oils, use of, for arousal, 43, 103
Oral-genital sex, 6, 30, 73, 82. *See also* Cunnilingus; Fellatio
  hygiene for, 82
  oils with, 43, 82
  positioning for, 82
Orgasm, 84
  cunnilingus, 83
  fantasizing of, 4, 70, 103

Paraplegia, defined, 103
Partner, assistance of
  in appliance removal, 27, 28, 30
  observing reactions of, 5
  in undressing, 27, 31
Penis
  erection of. *See* Erection, penile
  stimulation of, 46–47
  stroking of, 38
  stuffing technique, 53
Penis stiffener, use of, 68
Petting, 35
Pleasuring, 6
Positioning. *See under* Intercourse, sexual
Pregnancy, 4, 103
Preparation for sexual relations, difficulties in
  solving of, 27, 28
  use of aide in, 28

Quadriplegia, 105

Rectum, stimulation of, 48
Reflex erection. *See under* Erection, penile
Relationships, developing of, 3
Relaxation, after sexual arousal, 92
Reproduction
  attitudes toward, 5
  female and, capacity of, 4
  male and, capacity of, 4

Satisfaction, sexual, 5, 51
  attitudes necessary for, 6
  importance of, 5

Self-confidence, 96
Self-doubt, 95
　handling of, by communication, 96
Self-image
　projection of, 3
　related to sexuality, 2, 3
Sensation, mental transference of (sensory amplification), 3, 5, 99
Stimulation. *See also* Manual stimulation
　patterns of, 48–49
Stuffing technique, 53, 105

Talking. *See* Verbalization
Testicles, damage of, reproduction and, 4
Texas catheter, 22, 100
　putting on, 28
　removal of, 20
Touching, 35, 36
Trust, 2, 3

Undressing, assistance by partner in, 27, 31
Urine, leakage of, 24
Urine-collection appliances
　checking of, 26
　handling of, 22, 31
　leakage of, 24, 70
　for night-time use, 14
　positioning of, during intercourse, 14
　removal of, 20
　types of, 99

Vagina. *See also* Clitoris, manual stimulation of, 84
　stroking of, 38
Verbalization, arousal by, 35
Vibrators, for arousal, 38, 44, 88, 105

Water bed, use of, for sexual intercourse, 70
Wheelchair, use of, for sexual intercourse, 66